THE

Healthy Family

HANDBOOK

➤ ⬳

Natural
Remedies for
Parents and Children

THE
Healthy
Family
HANDBOOK

➤ ⬅

Natural
Remedies for
Parents and Children

by Louise Taylor & Lisa Marie Nelson
Foreword by Joseph E. Mitchell, D. C.

Charles E. Tuttle Co., Inc.
Boston ➤ Rutland, Vermont ⬅ Tokyo

This book presents information and material about alternative health treatments. The remedies presented here are intended to supplement, and not replace, treatment by a physician or other licensed medical practitioner. Consult your health care provider before adopting any of the treatments described herein. The adoption and application of the material offered in this book is at the reader's discretion and sole responsibility. The authors and publisher of this book are not responsible in any manner whatsoever for any injury that may occur indirectly or directly from the use of this book.

First published in 1997 by Charles E. Tuttle Co., Inc.
of Rutland, Vermont, and Tokyo, Japan, with editorial offices at
153 Milk Street, Boston, Massachusetts 02109

Library of Congress Cataloging-in-Publication Data

Taylor, Louise.
    The healthy family handbook : natural remedies for parents and children /
Louise Taylor and Lisa Marie Nelson.—1st ed.
        p. cm.
    Includes bibliographical references.
    ISBN 0-8048-3097-5
    1. Alternative medicine—Popular works. I. Nelson, Lisa Marie.
II. Title.
R733.T386 1997
615.5—dc20   96–45988
                                                                  CIP

First Edition
1 3 5 7 9 10 8 6 4 2   05 04 03 02 01 00 99 98 97

Book design by Jill Winitzer
Cover design by Kathryn Sky-Peck

Contents

List of Illustrations

Acknowledgments

To my gurus Babgawan Nitynanda and Guru Mayi Chidvilasananda, who always guide me on my spiritual journey and are my inspiration in writing, I give my heartfelt thanks. I would also like to express my thanks to my supporting staff, students, and friends at the Healing Arts Center, who always inspire me to take the concerns of the health of people one step further. I would like to add my appreciation to my family, who always support me in my dedication to health and the healing of people. —Louise Taylor

Many thanks to my family for their ever-present love and support. I have learned so much from my children. Parenting has opened up for me a whole new world of insight, inspiration, and opportunity. Thanks to my friends at CH.A.D.D. for their encouragement and enthusiasm. Thank you to Jennifer for her time and loyalty in helping get this all done, to Gina for making my life easier, and to Andy for his friendship and good advice. Much appreciation to Dr. Deepak Chopra and Dr. Brian Rees for guiding me toward health and bliss with Ayurveda, and to Dr. Joseph Mitchell, who teaches me so much about healing and helping. And a special thank you to Louise: my teacher, my mentor, my friend. —Lisa Marie Nelson

Foreword

It was with great pleasure that I had the opportunity to evaluate the manuscript of this book because it truly sheds light on a number of alternative health care remedies.

Alternative health care has been defined in many ways, and has given rise to considerable confusion, controversy, and misinformation. I consider it to be the treatment of disease or injury utilizing nutritional, herbal, physical, and many other methods not usually associated with western traditional medical practice and surgery. I suppose you could say that anything you do in the way of treating or preventing illness that is not routinely performed, prescribed, or provided by traditional medical doctors could be considered "alternative."

The medical profession has long considered any form of treatment that was not taught in medical school to be ineffective and often referred to anyone who recommended or prescribed such methods as a charlatan. As a chiropractic physician for the past thirty-five years I have been intimately involved with most of the various practices known as alternative healing. Chiropractic has always been a non-medical and non-surgical approach that uses natural methods in addition to the distinctly unique chiropractic spinal adjustment.

My partners and I use many of these alternative approaches on a daily basis in our practice. It is my experience that when these methods are used in combination, remarkable, and sometimes astounding, results are achieved. I have used and recommended that my patients take various preparations containing vitamins, minerals, and herbs. We have also recommended relaxation techniques, meditation, homeopathy, acupressure and acupuncture, various forms of exercise, and many Yoga techniques. I have seen dramatic results in patients with chronic conditions, such as high blood pressure, chronic headaches, sleeplessness, colds, influenza, dysmenorrhea, and many more.

As a practicing chiropractic physician I am not opposed to the use of pharmaceuticals and surgery when absolutely necessary. However, I believe that because of intensive advertising by pharmaceutical firms, many people have been led to believe that there is a pill for almost every symptom. When a patient comes to us with a condition that can be treated safely with natural methods, I believe we should avoid unnatural chemical compounds and, whenever possible, utilize these natural methods. Prevention is still, of course, the best cure of all.

As an example, during the last few years large numbers of the population have been placed on drugs like Prozac, which is used for the treatment of depression (among other things). As with any compound of that type there are side effects, and sometimes these can be devastating.

In our practice we have found that most patients who are using the herb St. John's Wort (sometimes combined with some other herbs), in combination with specific corrective spinal adjustments, have shown marked improvement in the symptoms of depression without the use of Prozac.

For many years, anyone who suggested using vitamin E and bioflavonoids (antioxidants that enhance vitamin C activity) as a preventative for coronary disease was ridiculed. Now, this treatment is often recommended by top cardiologists. In fact, one recent study published in the prestigious *British Medical Journal* (vol. 312, 1996, pp. 478-81) showed that lower than average dietary intake of bioflavonoids can increase the risk of coronary heart disease.

In the past, vitamins were usually considered unnecessary by traditional medical physicians, except in very rare instances, because traditional medical schools taught that people receive all "necessary" nutrition from a normal diet. Now it is becoming increasingly common for traditional medical doctors to recommend vitamin and mineral supplementation for many conditions.

Consumer interest in alternative medicine has increased to an all time high, and because of public pressure the United States Government set up a special office for the study of alternative treatment methods in 1992. The United States Department of Health and Human Services Office of Alternative Medicine has been mandated to provide scientifically valid and useful information to the public about alternative and complementary therapies. The American Medical Association has even commissioned a study to determine why so many Americans were seeking treatment from alternative care providers. Insurance companies are beginning to institute a more holistic approach to health care by developing plans for reimbursing alternative treatments, including most of the natural methods mentioned in this book.

It is always a pleasure to work with patients who have some knowledge of these alternative methods, so when Lisa Nelson came to me as a patient I found it refreshing to work with someone who was able to contribute to her own health and wellness through her knowledge and use of these alternative approaches.

I believe you will find that the information contained in this book can help you along the road to discovering new energy, vitality, and wellness in both mind and body. You will find valuable information about nine alternative health care options: acupressure, aromatherapy, Ayurveda, Bach Flowers, color therapy, herbal therapy, homeopathy, meditation, and Yoga. These alternative therapies often work synergistically and may be more powerful when used in combination. They are often helpful when used in conjunction with traditional therapies and may enhance the effects of the traditional methods. Sometimes alternative therapies are useful for alleviating some of the side effects of traditional medications.

In my practice, I treat each case as a unique individual. Even patients with apparently the same symptoms have a unique body chemistry and will respond differently to treatment. For this reason, we work with our patients to establish their individual needs, and later we work to help them maintain good health through various lifestyle changes and alternative treatments. Many of these are discussed in this book.

I encourage you to be aware of these alternative approaches to health care and to take an active interest in maintaining your own health and well-being. When mind and body are in balance, positive things are drawn to you. I believe this book can help you along the road to health and wellness.

Most important of all, allow your love to nourish you and all those near to you.

—Joseph E. Mitchell, D. C.

Preface

It's two o'clock in the morning and your child crawls into your bed. His feet are cold, his head is hot, and he just doesn't feel good. What do you do? Raid the medicine cabinet guessing at dosages? Get on the phone with the doctor's answering service? Spend the night in the emergency room?

Every parent has been in this situation; we certainly have. We want to do all that we can to help our children. But often we feel limited, powerless in the face of those symptoms at the beginning of many illnesses.

The truth is that there is quite a bit that we can do, on our own, to help our children and ourselves to heal and to be healthy. At the Healing Arts Center, people come in every day seeking advice about how to treat common health problems. They are surprised at all the over-the-counter, natural health products and treatment choices we present to them, many of which they never knew about before. Regardless of the course of action they choose, they feel better just knowing that they have some control and decision-making power regarding their own health care.

For parents, this control is even more important. Children look to their parents for solutions. It's frustrating when you can't make your own child feel better. But your hands aren't tied! Whether it's the sniffles, chicken pox, or a behavior problem, there are a myriad of simple, noninvasive, and natural ways in which you can address the problem and comfort your child. There are alternatives to sitting through a sleepless night waiting for the doctor to answer his or her page.

We highly recommend that you and your family design a healthy lifestyle routine that will improve the quality of all of your lives. In this book we have given you many ideas that you can use to incorporate healthy habits into your daily life.

This book is intended to empower you with some of the many alternative health care solutions you have for addressing your family's health problems. *It is very important for you to seek medical advice from your doctor, because the benefits of Western medicine cannot be denied.* If a child's illness persists for more than forty-eight hours or if he or she is running a fever or is in pain, please seek medical attention immediately. These alternative treatments and therapies are meant to be used in conjunction with your doctor's advice or when you can't get to your doctor right away. You also can use these remedies or techniques along with what your doctor has prescribed. In this way you will be contributing to your own well-being. Sometimes, for small problems and minor discomfort, a simple home health remedy is sufficient.

Combining two or more of the therapies that we suggest is very beneficial. You may need to experiment and come to your perfect combination of therapies by trial and error. There are, however, some techniques that will blend better with your individual lifestyle and needs, so you may want to choose one or more that fits your personality or that is more suitable for your family. We have found some combinations to be of particular value in our own families. These include the combination of Bach Flowers and acupressure (which Louise uses regularly in her healing practice), aromatherapy and Yoga, Ayurveda products along with color therapy (which Lisa Marie uses daily for her children and herself), homeopathy combined with Yoga, and herbs combined with aromatherapy. In many of these combinations, an energetic type of healing modality is coupled with body movement or a natural plant substance. Joining therapies from two different systems helps to enhance each of the individual systems.

One of the best things about at-home healing treatments is that by using them, you teach your children how to take care of themselves. We are raising a generation of wise, wonderful people who are interested in taking responsibility for their own health. *The Healthy Family Handbook* will give you fantastic resource material that will make you feel confident in treating yourself and your family naturally.

1

What's What—Explaining Age-Old Treatments Now New Again

It seems like people are really coming full circle now. After exploring our modern Western medical model, people are expressing a strong interest in getting back to ancient, more natural, noninvasive ways of dealing with illnesses. There are many different alternative systems of medicine from which to choose. Each has its own benefits; it's just a matter of which techniques you are comfortable using. Some people will respond better with certain forms of treatment, so just find out what you like and what works best for you.

In this book, we explore nine different kinds of alternative therapies to treat various ailments and promote health and longevity: acupressure, aromatherapy, Ayurveda, Bach Flowers, color therapy, herbs, homeopathy, meditation, and Yoga. You will find a combination of these therapies to be more beneficial than using them one at a time.

All of these therapies can be used as preventive measures to keep you and your family healthy because they keep the body balanced and energy flowing freely. They are also important as a part of your daily routine to enhance the quality of your life. These therapies help to alleviate emotional and other stress-related symptoms before they manifest as illnesses. Each of them also resolves symptoms that have already developed, bringing the body back into balance and relieving uncomfortable or nagging symptoms. We will present specific products within each of the systems that we have found to work most effectively on individual conditions.

✦ ACUPRESSURE ✦

Thousands of years before American and European scientists discovered atoms, electrons, and electricity, the Chinese developed a concept of the entire universe as being in balance between negative (*yin*) and positive (*yang*) energy forces. Yin and yang represent the negative and positive dualism existing within all things, from the protons and electrons of the atoms to the seasonal changes and all of the opposite or opposing forces in nature. This duality is fundamental in both ancient Chinese and modern scientific thought.

The ancient Chinese saw the human body as a microcosm of the universe; in order to function properly, the body, like the universe, requires a balance of yin and yang energy. Thousands of years ago these principles were written down in the *I Ching*, or *The Book of Changes*. It is not necessary to accept Chinese philosophical concepts in order to learn acupressure. (The actual meaning of acupressure is "finger pressure.") We can, however, use the formulas described in the 4,000-year-old text *The Yellow Emperor's Classic of Internal Medicine* for relieving pain and disability throughout the body.

The Chinese also developed the concept of "vital energy," which is called *chi*. This energy is even more subtle than electrical energy. The fundamental energy of the universe, it enters the human body through the breath and through food. Food and air then combine to form the life energy of all living beings.

Practitioners of Oriental medicine believe that vital energy has a definite, predictable route throughout the body. It flows along pathways that traverse the body in a fixed pattern somewhat like the network of a complex railway system. These pathways are divided into major routes called meridians, which are named for the organ or function they serve. On these routes are numerous tiny points called acupuncture, or acupressure, points where the energy comes to the surface of the body. It is interesting to note that a modern method of electronic photography, called Kirlian photography, now enables us to locate acupuncture/acupressure points precisely. Kirlian photographs have proved that the points are exactly where the ancient Chinese showed them to be. These points respond to any change in the flow of vital energy. They appear to act somewhat like resistors in an electrical current by adjusting the speed and power of the flow. The response is a kind of fluid elasticity that tightens or slackens as necessary. The vital energy reaches the organs through the meridians and acupressure points. If the organ or gland nourished by a particular flow is not functioning properly, points along the meridian will be painful or stiff. By reestablishing the energy flow along this pathway, the organ or gland will be revitalized and health will be restored. The meridians also can be thrown off balance by the tensions and stresses of modern life. When this happens, the flow of vital energy becomes blocked, too intense, or too weak, resulting in the development of disorders in body functioning.

A meridian that is low or deficient in energy must be stimulated to bring a fresh supply of energy to it. When a meridian is lacking energy, the organ involved, as well as the nearby muscles and nerves, is not working at peak performance. Ultimately this can have an adverse effect on the vitality of the entire body. Stimulating the specific point, depending on the ailment, will generate a revitalization of that particular energy flow and thereby remove blocks within the organ's meridian system that could prevent a state of good health.

⇢ AROMATHERAPY ⇠

Aromatherapy is the science of using the fragrance of essential plant oils in healing treatments. Plants have been used for their healing properties for thousands of years. In 4500 B.C., for example, Egyptians used perfumed oils derived from natural sources. They knew that the aromatic quality of plants and herbs could improve digestion, and they used spices in their cooking. Garlic also provided antibacterial properties and helped to prevent epidemics. According to a translation of the inscription on the Pyramid of Cheops, every morning each slave who worked to build the pyramid was given a clove of garlic because its aromatic properties would provide him with strength and good health. Now aromatherapy is used with great success all over the world.

Aromatherapy is an energetic healing technique that uses the vibratory energy of various aromas to shift the body's energy system and bring relief from physical symptoms. The aromas used are distilled directly from plants and placed in an oil base, forming what is called essential oils.

Two reasons for the popularity of aromatherapy are the ease with which the essential oils can be used and their wide variety of uses. They can be diluted with a neutral carrier oil and used for massage. When they're used in this way, the element of human contact is added, and that contact is always a benefit in healing treatments.

Essential oils can also be used in aromatic baths. By itself, bath water is soothing and therapeutic. When combined with essential oils, the soothing effect is enhanced.

Compresses can be made from essential oils, either hot or cold depending on the condition that is being treated. The oils also can be mixed in creams or lotions.

Essential oils are potent and should be used in moderation. The skin absorbs oils applied to it. When inhaled, fragrances have an effect on the mind, which has an effect on the body.

→ AYURVEDA ←

Translated from Sanskrit, *Ayurveda* means "science of life." Ayurvedic medicine is originally from India, where it has been around for over 5,000 years. Maharishi Mahesh Yogi, the founder of Transcendental Meditation, introduced Ayurveda to the West in the early 1980s. Because of the tremendous work and dedication of Dr. Deepak Chopra (medical doctor, lecturer, and bestselling author), Ayurveda has become popular and widely recognized in the United States as a valuable system of healing. Today many doctors combine Ayurveda and Western medicine in a harmonious blending of East and West.

The principle behind Ayurveda is balance. Ayurveda is used in two ways: as a preventive health care system by keeping the body balanced, and as a responsive health care system to bring the body back into balance. While Western medicine looks at an illness and seeks to rid the patient of its symptoms, Ayurveda looks at the whole patient and seeks to bring him or her back into a state of balance, thereby creating a natural state of health.

Mind/body balance is obtained through a connection between the mind and body, where thought acts on matter to create health or illness. In the place where mind meets body, there are three operating principles of nature, or *doshas: Vata, Pitta,* and *Kapha.* While we cannot see these doshas, we see the effect that they have on our minds and bodies. They operate as "metabolic principles." Each person is born with a unique combination of each of these three doshas, which make up his or her mind/body type. The goal is to find your particular mind/body type and keep it in balance for optimum health. This balance is achieved through proper diet, exercise, and lifestyle.

⤷ BACH FLOWERS ⬿

Bach Flowers are named for the late Edward Bach of England, a homeopathic doctor who discovered the thirty-eight flower remedies and their method of treatment. Dr. Bach believed that in this life we have two purposes: to work on our Divine Purpose (to grow spiritually) and to serve our fellow human beings. His theory was that if you are not doing both of these things, then disease can set in.

This system of healing is based on shifting the emotional energy of an individual through the vibrations found in specific flowers. The essence of these flowers has been potentized into drops that can be administered in a variety of ways. By shifting the vibratory energy connected with our emotions, our physical condition has been found to respond accordingly.

Rather than focus on the disease, Bach Flowers looks at the emotional state that is the root cause of disease. Under stress from a negative emotional state, the body loses its natural resistance to disease and gets sick much more easily. By correcting the emotional state, the disease will have nowhere to flourish and will naturally go away. In Dr. Bach's own words, "There is no true healing unless there is a change in outlook, peace of mind, and inner happiness."

All of our moods and reactions fall into seven basic emotional states. They are

1. Fear
2. Uncertainty
3. Insufficient interest in present circumstances
4. Loneliness
5. Oversensitivity to influences and ideas
6. Despondency or despair
7. Overcare for welfare of others

The thirty-eight Bach Flower remedies each facilitate emotional correction in one of these categories.

→ COLOR THERAPY ←

Color therapy is an energy system that directly infuses a particular energy vibration into the body to shift the body's vibratory energy.

Color is an important part of our everyday lives. We use it to decorate our homes and we wear it in our clothing. Color is also a part of our health. When someone is sad, we say they're "blue." When they're feeling fine, they're "in the pink." When we feel angry, we "see red." And optimists are often accused of looking at the world through "rose-colored glasses." When harnessed, the energy of color is an effective and powerful healing tool.

There are seven colors of the rainbow: red, orange, yellow, green, blue, indigo, and violet.

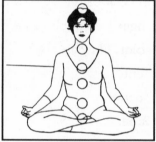

In the body, there are seven *chakras*, or energy centers. Each chakra corresponds with one of the seven colors. By keeping the chakras in balance, the body is kept in balance and is healthy.

The first chakra is at the base of the spine. It corresponds with red. Red is traditionally associated with strength, vigor, sexual love, danger, and charity.

Near the top of the lumbar area of the back is the second chakra, which corresponds with orange. Orange is associated with happiness, adaptability, attraction, plenty, and kindness.

The third chakra is located near the solar plexus and corresponds with yellow. Yellow is associated with mental effort, charm, confidence, persuasion, joy, and comfort.

The fourth chakra is near the heart, and it corresponds with green. Green is associated with health, wealth, luck, fertility, energy, and growth.

The fifth chakra is in the throat and corresponds with blue. Blue is associated with communication, understanding, tranquility, truth, devotion, sincerity, health, and patience.

In the middle of the forehead is the sixth chakra, which corresponds with indigo. Indigo is associated with ambition, depression, changeability, impulsiveness, and dignity.

The seventh chakra is at the top of the head, and it corresponds with violet. Violet is associated with spirituality, sentimentality, power, and sadness.

Generally speaking, in color therapy, warm colors (reds and oranges) are used to stimulate. Restaurants and hotels often use these colors in their decor because they are known to stimulate the appetite. Cool colors (blues and greens) are used to calm. Hospitals and doctors' offices frequently use these colors to make people feel more at peace in their surroundings.

Individuals who use color for natural healing expose themselves to colored lights, envision a particular color through meditation, or create an environment using colors. These techniques and many others can be used to treat illness.

✦ HERBS ✦

Herbs have been used for thousands of years because of their potent healing properties. Most traditional medicines are derived from specific herbs. In their natural state, herbs can have a whole-body effect in treating symptoms, enabling people to avoid using the stronger medicines prescribed by doctors. Herbs are a gentler form of medicine and therefore have fewer side effects than prescribed medications or over-the-counter drugs. While herbs may be slower in their action, they also encourage the body to heal itself more naturally.

Herbs are natural and work to strengthen the body. There are many different kinds of herbs, and each serves a different function: some fight infection, some help digestion, some are relaxing, and so on. Herbal medicine, or *naturopathy,* is becoming more popular today as people discover that plant-based medicine is a safe, gentle, effective, and practical means of self-care.

Herbs help the body in many ways. They cleanse, regulate body functions, provide nutrition, increase the body's energy level, and stimulate the immune system. They can be made into teas, added to foods, or taken as tablets. The potency of tablets varies with the manufacturer, so users should be sure to read the dosage on the bottle. Herbs may be taken singly but often work more effectively in combination.

→ HOMEOPATHY ←

Homeopathic medicine was developed in the early 1800s by Dr. Samuel Hahnemann of Germany. It is a natural pharmaceutical science and is known as an energetic medical system since it uses minute doses of natural substances (animal, vegetable, and mineral) to stimulate the body's own defenses.

Homeopathy is a word derived from the Greek *homoios,* which means "similar," and *pathos,* which means "disease." It is medicine based on the law of similars. This principle says that a substance will help to heal symptoms similar to those that it is known to cause. This is the same principle behind immunization. Homeopathy is also known as a medicine of similars.

The choice of homeopathic medicine is determined by a person's unique symptoms. Each person is different, each disease is different, and each remedy depends on the combination of symptoms for that person. Whether you are seeing a homeopathic doctor or self-prescribing, you must look for your unique symptoms when determining the medication you need.

→ MEDITATION ←

For centuries Eastern cultures have used many meditation practices to expand and circulate energy throughout the mind and body. These Eastern traditions believe that the individual's consciousness is a single manifestation of a larger universal consciousness or energy that exists everywhere and in everything.

Further, they believe that because the human mind is restless and seldom still, a veil is formed that brings about sensesations of separateness and limitation. Through the process of meditation, which stills and calms the mind, inner boundaries slowly dissolve bringing about a heightened state of identification with the universal consciousness. This, in turn, produces a feeling of profound contentment, relaxation, and fulfillment.

Many recent scientific studies, in the East and West alike, have explored the effects of regular meditation practices. An impressive body of documentation indicates that when the meditator's mind and body transcend the limitations of moment-to-moment consciousness, a state of balance and centeredness is achieved. By decreasing the amount of internal and external stimuli that must be responded to, the body's metabolism is lowered. Additionally, as cellular activity throughout the body slows, the need for oxygen is reduced, while the increase in relaxation permits an increased flow of blood to the muscles, which decreases the heart's workload. Finally, during meditation the cells of the brain fire in a synchronous manner, fostering integrated functioning between lower and higher brain centers and between left and right hemispheres.

Meditation ultimately provides a profound sense of inner silence and tranquillity, freeing the meditator from pressure, concern, tension, and anxiety. By decreasing these limiting states, people who meditate have additional energy to use in more positive ways.

Most forms of meditation involve three principles or inner activities: (1) reflection and focused thought, (2) receptiveness and quietness, and (3) creation and formulation.

Reflection and Focused Thought

There is already a strong element of meditation in everyone's life. When you focus your mind on a story you are reading, or when you are studying something that you wish to know, you are concentrating on one thing to the exclusion of all other distractions. This is similar to meditation, where your focus is on quieting your mind. Through the power of concentration or focused thought, you can accomplish great things, and the same is true for meditation.

Meditation also arises spontaneously when you focus your attention on a specific object or person, such as a child at play, a beautiful place, or a favorite painting.

When your mind focuses outside, it perceives the outer world.

When you begin to look within, it discovers the beauty and tranquillity of the inner world.

Receptiveness and Quietness

The stillness and quietness you experience when in a state of meditation provide a deep rest for both your mind and body. Because your nervous system is allowed a period of recuperation, one that can be even more beneficial than a restful night's sleep, you will notice an increase in your energy level each time you meditate. You will be awake and alert during hours of activity. Meditation before bed allows the mind and body to prepare for sleep and will help you to drift off easily.

When you meditate, you also become more open to the intuitive part of your mind, which enables you to be more aware of your needs, gives inspiration, and even provides solutions to unresolved problems.

Meditation helps children learn to focus and to quiet their minds and bodies. It allows them time with themselves to discover their inner nature.

Creation and Formulation

By learning to focus uncritically on one thing at a time while you meditate, you develop a kind of self-discipline that increases your self-awareness. With practice, you can better understand and accept habitual patterns of perception, thought, and feeling that previously had influenced your life without your complete awareness.

Through meditation you are able to go beyond your identification with the body and discover that you have an existence that is quite apart from your tensions and physical problems. You are also able to go beyond the mind by realizing that you are not your thoughts but the witness of those thoughts as they come and go.

You learn that your true identity is within the inner stillness, within the peace and satisfaction that is your own consciousness. When you have achieved that realization, you can use meditation to experience the powerful energies of imagination, visualization, and clear formulation of goals that ultimately bring about more positive and desirable life experiences.

→ YOGA ←

Yoga originated in India more than 6,000 years ago. Practiced by Tibetan monks, the techniques and theories were initially handed down orally from teachers to students. Later they were written down. The first written account is attributed to the Indian sage Patanjali, who codified the complete system of Yoga in the second century B.C. In the Yoga Sutras, which remain very important in India to this day, Patanjali describes eighty-four main Yoga postures from the thousands then in use. These same postures are basic to the study of Yoga in India today.

The word *Yoga* is derived from the Sanskrit root verb *yuj*, which means "to join" or "to unite." It signifies the joining of the individual with the universal reality. It also means the union of the conscious mind with the deeper levels of the unconscious, which results in a totally integrated personality. Just as acupressure and Ayurvedic practices seek perfect balance in the human body, the yogic ideal of unification is called *mukusha* and connotes a perfect balance or state of naturalness. Every living being strives toward this ideal, which is described in the Christian religion as "the peace which passeth all understanding." When people begin to search for balance and natural harmony in their own lives, they begin to grow on a path that leads to deeper understanding and fulfillment. At such a time they learn that satisfaction comes from something that they find deep within and does not rely on external stimulation. In the sixth chapter of the *Bhagavad Gita,* the textbook of Yoga philosophy, Yoga is explained as meaning a deliverance from the sorrows of this world:

> When his mind, intellect and self are under control, freed from restless desire, so that they rest in the spirit within, a man becomes a Yukta—one in communion with God. A lamp does not flicker in a place where no winds blow; so it is with a Yogi, who controls his mind, intellect and self, being absorbed in the spirit within him. When the restlessness of the mind, intellect and self is stilled through the practice of Yoga, the Yogi, by the grace of the spirit within himself, finds fulfillment. Then he knows the joy eternal which is beyond the pale of the senses which his reason cannot grasp. He abides in this reality and moves not therefrom. He has found the treasure above all others. There is nothing higher than this. He who has achieved it shall not be moved by the greatest sorrow.

This is the real meaning of Yoga—a deliverance from contact with pain and sorrow.

Although balance is basic to all existence, it is often upset. Yoga attempts to restore it through a threefold path of development: physical, mental, and spiritual. Yoga teaches that there is no artificial separation between that which is body and that which is mind. The goal is to gain control of the body's energy flow and to direct it in positive, healing ways. The vital energy called *chi* by the Chinese and *ki* by the

Japanese is called *prana* in India. Prana is seen to be everywhere and in everything; it is the basic force that animates all matter. In the study of Yoga, the life force, or prana, is closely associated with breathing practices that control and direct this important energy. Freed and able to flow throughout the body, it can stimulate both body and mind; when it is blocked and distorted, you may feel sapped and depleted.

The Yoga postures, called *asanas,* and breathing techniques combine to provide vitality and well-being. Each of the postures is enhanced by the addition of proper breathing (*Pranayama*). The stretches, breathing techniques, and deep-relaxation exercises balance and tone the entire body. They provide an effective method for dealing with today's fast-paced lives and give quick and observable results in relieving stress and tension. In addition, Yoga is fun for the whole family.

2

Getting Started—The Basics

Now you know what all of these disciplines are. So how can you put them to use in your own home? The first thing to do is to have the materials you need handy. Then you've got to change your habits a little bit. When you have a headache, for example, instead of reaching for the old aspirin, look to see what your options are, what you have available, and then experiment to find out which remedy works best for you.

Remember, it is important to seek traditional medical advice first. The natural remedies described in this book can be used for at-home care, or they can be used to complement other medical treatments. We strongly recommend that you see your medical doctor for any medical condition. By using natural remedies in addition to medical care, you can set yourself on a journey of effective self-care and self-discovery. The benefits are age-old, the rewards are many.

We have found that combining holistic therapies, such as aromatherapy with Yoga, Bach flower remedies with acupressure, and Ayurveda products with color therapy, increases their effectiveness. Experiment to find the combinations that work best for your family.

❖ ACUPRESSURE ❖

The tools for acupressure are your fingers, so you always have the necessary equipment with you. Be sure your fingernails are short so that they do not poke into your skin. The only other things you need are the information and illustrations provided in this book. When using acupressure, firm, even pressure, consistency, and the accurate location of the points make all the difference in the quality of the results.

Be sure to stimulate the points on both the right and left sides of the body or directly on the midline of the body, either while sitting or while lying down.

Do not press on the body in any area that is injured or any place where the skin is broken.

Press the acupressure points for 1 to 2 minutes each, repeating 3 to 4 times daily. It is easy for people of all ages—even children—to use these points on themselves, but the pressure should be firm and steady. We suggest that parents stimulate these points on themselves as their children press their own pressure points. Working in this way will encourage children as well as teach them correct methods.

❖ AROMATHERAPY ❖

Aromatherapy is so versatile that you can use it just about anytime, anywhere. All you need to get started are the essential oils, which are readily available at health food stores and some pharmacies. You can dab a few drops of an essential oil on a cotton ball and carry it with you throughout your busy day. You can keep a bottle of essential oils in your desk. When you're feeling tired or stressed, just add a few drops to a bowl of hot water and breathe in the fragrance.

Children can carry a cotton ball in a pocket or backpack. Kids especially like the aromas of cinnamon and vanilla.

An electric diffuser is a convenient way to use aromatherapy. Simply fill the diffuser about halfway with water and add a few drops of essential oil. Then plug in the diffuser. As the water heats, the aroma wafts gently through the room. Keep an eye on the water level so that it doesn't all evaporate and cause a hazard.

Light rings have become popular tools for aromatherapy users. They consist of a round "channel" ring with a gutter that fits over the top of a lighbulb. The rings usually are made of clay or aluminum. You put a few drops of essential oil in the gutter and set the ring on the lightbulb. When the light is on, the heat releases the aroma and the room is filled with fragrance. You can use this technique anytime you want to brighten your day in more ways than one!

Aroma "pots" are another easy way to use aromatherapy. These are tiny clay containers with a little cork in the top. You put a few drops of oil into the pot and keep the pot wherever you want a subtle hint of scent: in the car, at your desk, or in your closet. You should use separate pots for different oils, as the clay absorbs the fragrance.

Use essential oils for massage by diluting them in a carrier oil, such as the safflower, sunflower, or sesame oils you find in the supermarket. Use 2 drops of an essential oil for every 2 ounces of carrier oil. You can use essential oils to make an aromatic bath by dropping 2 to 3 drops in the water. Other ways to use the oils include in fragrant potpourris, or misted directly into the air with a perfume mister.

Throughout the book, we suggest different aromatherapies for different conditions. As the following four essential oils are used again and again, you may want to keep them on hand at all times:

→ **Chamomile**

→ **Lavender**

→ **Peppermint**

→ **Thyme**

See Appendix 2, the Resources section, to find some sources for obtaining essential oils.

→ AYURVEDA ←

An Ayurvedic physician can provide the most accurate diagnosis of a mind/body type. Typically, the doctor will use a special pulse diagnosis, have you answer a series of questions, and look at your tongue and your physical features to determine your particular combination of doshas. The doctor can also detect any imbalances and recommend specific Ayurvedic herbs and lifestyle adjustments, if necessary. If you are interested in learning more about Ayurveda and adopting this lifestyle, and particularly if you are not feeling well, it would be a good idea to consult an Ayurvedic professional.

Vata, Pitta, and Kapha doshas are present in everyone, just in different combinations. And all three doshas need to be kept in balance. To do so, you need to be aware of your own mind/body type. Your mind/body type is determined by which dosha or doshas are most prevalent in your personality and physical makeup.

The following test will help you to learn more about yourself and discover your own mind/body type. For each of the questions, read the statement and answer from 0 to 4 how true each one is for you. Answer 0 if it is not true at all. Answer 4 if it is very true.

Write down and total your score for each section, then compare your scores for each mind/body type at the end. Parents should work with their children to make sure they understand the questions and to help add up the scores. The three scores should give you a good idea about your type. The highest score determines your predominant dosha and thus your mind/body type. Sometimes one dosha will be obviously dominant, but often two doshas are equally prominent. In this case, the higher score is your dominating dosha, but the second dosha is also important in understanding your mind/body type. While all three doshas express themselves in some way in everyone, in both body and personality, usually one or two are dominant and need more attention to maintain balance.

VATA	Not True at All			Very True	
I don't like cold weather	0	1	2	3	4
I don't gain weight easily	0	1	2	3	4
I often become anxious and restless	0	1	2	3	4
My moods change quickly	0	1	2	3	4
I am creative, imaginative	0	1	2	3	4
I walk quickly	0	1	2	3	4
I have difficulty falling or staying asleep	0	1	2	3	4
I tend to make and change friends	0	1	2	3	4
I learn quickly and forget quickly	0	1	2	3	4
I become constipated easily	0	1	2	3	4
Under stress, I am easily excited	0	1	2	3	4
I have an irregular appetite	0	1	2	3	4
My skin tends to be dry, rough, especially in winter	0	1	2	3	4
My feet and hands tend to be cold	0	1	2	3	4
My hair tends to be dry	0	1	2	3	4

Vata Total _____

PITTA	**Not True at All**			**Very**	**True**
I don't like hot weather	0	I	2	3	4
My weight is average for my build	0	I	2	3	4
I tend to become intense, irritable	0	I	2	3	4
My moods are intense and change slowly	0	I	2	3	4
I am intelligent, efficient, a perfectionist	0	I	2	3	4
I have a determined walk	0	I	2	3	4
I sleep well, for an average length of time	0	I	2	3	4
Most of my friends are work-related	0	I	2	3	4
I have a good general memory	0	I	2	3	4
I have very regular bowel habits	0	I	2	3	4
Under stress, I am easily angered, critical	0	I	2	3	4
I am uncomfortable skipping meals	0	I	2	3	4
My skin is soft, ruddy	0	I	2	3	4
I like cold foods and drinks	0	I	2	3	4
My hair is fine, thin, reddish, or prematurely gray	0	I	2	3	4

Pitta Total: ———————

KAPHA	**Not True at All**			**Very**	**True**
I don't like damp, cool weather	0	I	2	3	4
I gain weight easily	0	I	2	3	4
I can be slow or depressed	0	I	2	3	4
My moods are mostly steady	0	I	2	3	4
My mind is calm, steady, stable	0	I	2	3	4
My walk is slow and steady	0	I	2	3	4
I generally sleep long and soundly	0	I	2	3	4
My friendships are long-lasting, sincere	0	I	2	3	4
I have a good long-term memory	0	I	2	3	4
I eat and digest slowly	0	I	2	3	4
I am stubborn, not easily ruffled	0	I	2	3	4
I can skip meals easily	0	I	2	3	4
My skin is oily, moist	0	I	2	3	4
I have good stamina, steady energy level	0	I	2	3	4

Kapha Total: ———————

Comparative Totals: VATA ———— **PITTA** ———— **KAPHA** ————

Every person is born with a unique balance of each of the three doshas. Generally one or two of the doshas will dominate, and this will determine the Ayurvedic routine for your mind/body type.

Chart 2.1 shows the characteristics of Vata, Pitta, and Kapha.

Refer to this table to compare your mind/body type with your own observations about yourself.

Vata

Vata-type people are generally thin and find it hard to gain weight. Because of this, Vatas have very little energy reserve and can tire easily and get themselves out of balance. Vatas need to get sufficient rest and not overdo things, stay warm, and keep a regular lifestyle routine.

The Vata dosha controls all movement in the body, including breathing, digestion, and nerve impulses from the brain. When Vata is out of balance, anxiety and other nervous disorders may be present. Digestive problems, constipation, cramps, and even premenstrual pain usually are attributed to a Vata imbalance.

The most important thing to know about Vata is that it leads the other doshas. Vata usually goes out of balance first, which causes the early stages of disease. More than half of all illnesses are Vata disorders. Balancing Vata is important for everyone, because when Vata is in balance, Pitta and Kapha are generally in balance as well.

Pitta

Pitta-type people are generally of medium size and well proportioned. They have a medium amount of physical energy and stamina.

	VATA	**PITTA**	**KAPHA**
Function:	Controls Movement	Controls Metabolism	Controls Structure
Key Word:	"Changeable"	"Intense"	"Relaxed"
Governs:	Colon	Intestines	Chest
Properties	Cold, Dry, Light, Rough	Hot, Light, Sharp, Moist	Cold, Heavy, Wet, Sticky
Composed of:	Air (& Space)	Fire (& Water)	Water (& Earth)
Aggravated by (Avoid):	• Wind • Caffeine • Traveling • Irregular routine • Irregular meals • Cold, dry weather • Excessive mental work	• Heat • Alcohol • Smoking • Pressure • Stress • Excessive spicy or salty foods • Excessive activity	• Cold • Damp • Oversleeping • Overeating • Heavy foods • Too little variety in life
Diet To Keep in Balance, Favor:	*Tastes:* • Sweet • Sour • Salty • Warm foods	*Tastes:* • Sweet • Astringent • Bitter • Cool foods (not cold)	*Tastes:* • Bitter • Pungent • Astringent • Warm, light foods
Digestion Tends to Be:	Variable, delicate	Strong, intense	Slow, heavy
Recommended Exercise for Balance:	*Activities:* Low-impact: • Yoga • Walking • Dancing	*Activities:* Competitive or team sports: • Baseball • Tennis Or cooling sports: • Swimming	*Activities:* Stimulating, regular exercise: • Body building • Running
Season:	Nov.-Feb. (Cold & Dry)	July-Oct. (Hot)	March-June (Cold & Wet)
Color to Balance:	Green	Blue	Red
When in Balance You Are:	• Enthusiastic • Alert • Flexible • Creative • Talkative • Responsive	• Loving • Content • Intelligent • Articulate • Courageous	• Affectionate • Steady • Methodical • High stamina • Resistant to illnesses
When Out of Balance You Are:	• Restless • Fatigued • Constipated • Anxious • Underweight	• Perfectionist • Frustrated • Angry • Impatient • Irritable • Prematurely gray or have early hair loss	• Dull • Prone to oily skin • Prone to allergies • Possessive • Apt to oversleep • Overweight

Chart 2.1 Ayurvedic Mind/Body Type Characteristics (The Three Doshas)

They also tend to be intelligent and have a sharp wit and a good ability to concentrate.

Fire is a characteristic of Pitta, whether it shows up as fiery red hair or a short temper. Since Pittas' body temperature is generally warm, Pitta types can go out of balance with overexposure to the sun. Their eyes are sensitive to light. They are ambitious by nature but also can be demanding and abrasive.

Pitta types are known for their strong digestion but should be careful not to abuse it. Their heat makes them particularly thirsty, and they should take caution not to douse their *agni,* or digestive fire, with too much liquid during meals.

Pitta dosha leads us to crave moderation and purity. We rely on Pitta to regulate our intake of food, water, and air. Any toxins, such as alcohol or tobacco, show up as a Pitta imbalance. Toxic emotions such as jealousy, intolerance, and hatred should also be avoided to keep Pitta in balance for optimum health.

Kapha

Kapha-type people tend to have sturdy, heavy frames, providing a good reserve of physical strength and stamina. This strength gives Kaphas a natural resistance to disease and a generally positive outlook about life.

The Kapha dosha is slow, and Kapha types tend to be slow eaters with slow digestion. They also speak slowly. They are calm and affectionate but, when out of balance, can become stubborn and lazy. They learn slowly, with a methodical approach, but also retain information well with a good understanding of it.

Kapha dosha controls the moist tissues of the body, so a Kapha imbalance may show up as a cold, allergies, or asthma. This is worse in Kapha season, March through June. Cold and wet weather aggravates Kapha.

Kapha types need to progress to stay in balance. They should not dwell in the past or resist change. They need lots of exercise and need to be careful not to overeat. Kaphas need stimulation to bring out their vitality. Kapha dosha teaches us steadiness and a sense of well-being.

Besides diet and exercise, there are four other Ayurvedic considerations for maintaining balance: the calendar, the clock, daily massage, and meditation.

Calendar

Weather and seasonal changes affect our balance. Everyone can benefit from adapting his or her routine to the season. Although seasonal changes vary in different parts of the country, the description for the Ayurvedic calendar remains the same. November through February, when the weather is typically cold and dry, is Vata season. When wind, cold, and dry weather continues, Vata accumulates in the environment, which can cause a Vata imbalance in the body. During this season, it is a good idea to adopt a more Vata diet and routine to keep Vata in balance. Stay warm, eat warm foods, and don't wear yourself out.

Pitta season comes during the summer, July through October, when the weather is hot. To keep Pitta in balance during this time, eat cool foods, such as salads. Drink cool, not ice-cold, liquids and avoid too much sun.

March through June is Kapha season, when it is cold and wet. This is the time you are more likely to get a cold from a Kapha imbalance.

Stay warm, eat light meals, and get enough regular exercise to help keep Kapha in balance.

Clock

Just as the seasons have attributes of the doshas, so do the hours of the day. At sunrise, or about 6:00 A.M., the day's cycle begins with Kapha. To take advantage of the Kapha cycle, it is best to awaken between 6:00 A.M. and 8:00 A.M. On awakening, you feel slow, relaxed, calm: all Kapha attributes. Kapha lasts until about 10:00 A.M. Even young children can reap the benefits of the Kapha hours by arising at sunrise.

From 10:00 A.M. to 2:00 P.M., it is Pitta time. You are at your most active and efficient during these hours. At noon, or lunchtime, your appetite is at its peak. Eat lunch between noon and 1:00 P.M. to use Pitta to your advantage. Lunch also should be your largest meal of the

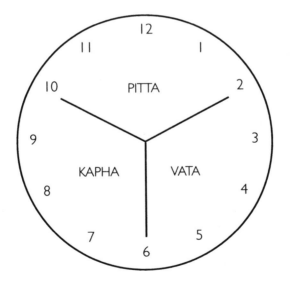

Chart 2.2 The Ayurvedic Daily Clock

day. Parents should pack nutritious snacks and lunches for children that include the best foods for their particular mind/body type. This is the best time for children to take tests in school, and it is their most productive learning time.

From 2:00 P.M. to 6:00 P.M. is Vata time, when you are most alert and creative. A light dinner should be eaten before 6:00 P.M., if possible, to take advantage of this energy.

The cycle repeats again in the evening hours. From 6:00 P.M. to 10:00 P.M. is Kapha time. Sunset brings the body rest and a slower pace. It is best to get to bed by 10:00 P.M. to take advantage of the natural Kapha rhythm of this time. For best digestion, eat dinner at least three hours before bedtime. Younger children who need more sleep should go to bed earlier so that they will still arise at sunrise.

Pitta time is 10:00 P.M. to 2:00 A.M., when Pitta keeps the body warm; the body also uses the Pitta heat to digest food and rebuild body tissue.

Vata time occurs again at 2:00 A.M. to 6:00 A.M. Vata creativity is expressed as active dreams. At this time, brain impulses are at their most active for the night.

Ayurvedic Massage (Abhyanga)

Ayurvedic massage offers many benefits. If done in the morning, it helps you to start your day off relaxed, which is essential in maintaining balance. When done at night, it promotes a restful night's sleep. It doesn't matter when you choose to do the massage, but you will receive the optimum benefits if you do it every day. Since the quality of Vata is dry and cold, a warm and oily massage provides an ideal balance for Vata types, though all types will notice increased health and vitality, especially during Vata season. The massage soothes the nervous system and the endocrine system, since skin produces endocrine hormones. It rejuvenates the skin, promoting a youthful appearance. It also eliminates toxins and tones the muscles. Parents can massage younger children and show older children how to do the massage themselves.

Sesame oil is recommended for Ayurvedic massage because it helps to balance all three of the doshas. It should be light oil and cured. (You can purchase cured oil or you can cure it yourself by heating the oil almost to boiling briefly and then cooling it down again.) The entire massage only requires about 2 ounces of oil.

Before you begin, warm the oil to skin temperature. The easiest way to do this is to keep a small plastic squeeze bottle filled with oil, and set the bottle in a bowl or cup of very hot water. Wait a few minutes for the oil to reach skin temperature.

While the oil warms, lay out a towel to protect the carpet or floor from any oil that may spill.

When you are ready, start the massage at your head. Drizzle a small amount of oil onto your scalp and massage it in with the palms of your hands. Use a clockwise, circular motion. Then gently massage your face and ears. If you have oily skin, avoid those areas that are prone to breakouts. Massaging the ears is excellent for balancing Vata.

Drizzle some oil on your palms and massage your neck, then move to your shoulders. Use a circular motion on your joints—shoulders, elbows, knees—and long up-and-down strokes on your limbs.

Be gentle on your torso. Use large, clockwise motions to massage the chest and stomach area.

Reach around to massage your back as best you can without straining.

Then massage your legs, ankles, and knees. Using the palms of your hands, vigorously massage your feet.

It is best to leave the oil on your body for 20 minutes before washing it off in a warm, not hot, shower or bath. You can use this time to meditate or do your Yoga exercises. If you don't have time to wait, that's fine. It's much better to do a quick massage than none at all. This is Lisa Marie's favorite part of her daily Ayurvedic routine.

Meditation

Ayurvedic medicine recommends transcendental meditation, which originated in India and was introduced to the West by Maharishi Mahesh Yogi. Transcendental meditation uses a combination of silence followed by mantra meditation—focusing on a word or phrase—and a period of silence again. The goal is to "transcend" the physical body and be in a place of calm all-knowingness. Transcendental meditation is taught one-on-one with an experienced teacher who gives you your mantra. Transcendental meditation classes can help you to understand and practice this discipline more effectively. For more information, see the Resources section.

Whichever meditation you choose, Ayurveda recommends that you practice 20 to 30 minutes in the morning and another 20 to 30 minutes in the evening. Time spent in silence or with nature helps keep the doshas in balance and can greatly improve your health and outlook on life. Ayurvedic researchers have found that meditation increases longevity and quality of life and can actually reverse the aging process.

✦ BACH FLOWERS ✦

Bach Flower remedies, which come in small bottles, are extremely concentrated. They are the energy vibrations from various flowers that have been distilled and concentrated. They come diluted in water to which a bit of alcohol has been added as a preservative. When kept tightly sealed, the remedies have an extremely long shelf life.

Bach Flower remedies can be used in several different ways. Adults can take 4 drops straight out of the bottle in their concentrated form and drop them under the tongue. Children can take 2 drops in the same fashion.

The most common way to take Bach Flower remedies is by diluting the concentrate in water and then drinking the water. If you are using just one flower, mix 4 drops of that flower in 1 ounce of water, then take 4 drops of the solution as often as needed. When diluted in water, the drops are really tasteless, so even picky children won't complain. If you are using a combination of flowers, mix 4 drops of each flower (up to a total of no more than six flowers) in 1 ounce of water, then take 4 drops of that solution as needed. You may want to purchase a dropper bottle that you can fill with water and then add the prescribed remedies. You can carry this bottle along with you and take drops throughout the day, either straight or by diluting the mixture further in a glass of water, tea, or juice. They will still have the desired effect.

A diluted Bach Flower remedy mixture can be spritzed directly into the air to alter the energy of a room. This is an especially effective way to experience the benefits of Bach Flowers.

Another way to use Bach Flowers is to drop some of the remedy onto your skin and massage it into the afflicted area. They can be worn like a perfume for emotional concerns. People of any age can sniff the fumes from the bottle for 30 seconds for a quick pick-me-up. You also can use them in your bath. Simply add 6 to 8 drops of the prescribed remedy to your or your children's bath water.

You can administer Bach Flowers to your children before they go to school in the morning, when they get home from school, at dinnertime, and before bed. By scheduling the doses in this way, you will increase compliance, as the children will not have to take the drops during their school day.

Throughout the books we mention various Bach Flower remedies for different ailments. A few seem to be used more commonly than others, and you may want to keep these on hand:

→ **Crab Apple**
→ **Olive**
→ **Rescue Remedy**
→ **Rescue Remedy cream**
→ **White Chestnut**

→ COLOR THERAPY ←

Color therapy is most effective when applied in the form of light. Hardware stores usually sell colored lightbulbs. These are excellent for use in healing. Get a chrome light reflector. It looks like a mixing bowl with a light socket at the bottom. The shiny surface reflects the colored light and helps to concentrate the light on the affected area.

Colored gels made from cellophane, found in art supply stores, are also a good way to make use of the healing power of light. You can tape the gel up to a sunny window and let the color shine through. The light source does not have to be the sun; you can fasten the gel over a regular lamp or use it in front of a slide projector.

Silk scarves can be draped over a lampshade to provide a glow of color.

Candles, of course, are an excellent source of color. You can buy colored candles or set white candles in colored glass.

You also can make color-infused water by placing a glass of water under a colored gel and setting it in the sun or under a lamp for an hour. When you drink the water, your body is filled with the vibrations of that color. Kids enjoy making these "potions," and color-infused water is a very powerful way to take in color vibrations.

Our children love to take colored baths. You can buy colored bath products at health stores. Do not use food coloring for baths, because it stains.

It is nice to have something available in each of the seven colors of the rainbow—red, orange, yellow, green, blue, indigo, and violet—for use whenever color therapy is needed. Try to have the following items in the various colors:

+ **Lightbulbs**
+ **Plastic or cellophane gels**
+ **Drinking glasses**
+ **Candles in a variety of colors**
+ **Color baths**

→ HERBS ←

A fun way to begin using herbs at home is to start an herb garden, either outdoors or on a sunny windowsill. Herbs are beautiful and fragrant and relatively easy to grow. Children can participate in gardening and learn from the experience.

Herbs are available in a variety of forms. You can buy them in bulk and make a tea by simmering them in water. You also can buy herbs in tea-bag form. Tea is the most potent form of herbal remedy. Powdered herbs that are placed into capsules or pressed into tablets are also available. This method is more convenient and may be preferred by those who do not like the taste of herb teas. If you use tablets or capsules, be aware that the potency varies with each manufacturer, so be sure to read the dosage on the bottle. Some herbs also come in liquid form. These may be diluted in water or juice to make them more palatable.

Herbs have a fairly long shelf life. Be sure to check for an expiration date on the bottle of any liquid herbs.

You can purchase herbal preparations at a health food store or order them from the Healing Arts Center. (See Appendix 2.)

Herbs may be taken singly, but they often work more effectively in combination.

The following herbs are beneficial for many symptoms. You may want to have some capsules of each on hand.

- → **Aloe vera**
- → **Chamomile**
- → **Echinacea**
- → **Ginger**
- → **Passionflower**
- → **Valerian**

→ HOMEOPATHY ←

Homeopathy, the medicine of similars, is a very specific science. When using homeopathy, you have to look carefully at all of your symptoms. If you misdiagnose yourself and take the wrong remedy, it probably will have no effect at all. But don't think that homeopathy doesn't work. You should just go back to the drawing board and rediagnose yourself. Chances are, you overlooked something that could make a difference in deciding which remedy to take. If you don't get the results you're looking for within one or two tries, consult a homeopathic physician in your area.

Homeopathy is a safe and powerful tool in treating a variety of ailments. The trick is to find the specific remedy for your particular condition. The most important tool in self-diagnosing is one of the many books on homeopathy. These books are like encyclopedias in which you can find specific combinations of symptoms and correlate them to the appropriate homeopathic remedy. Two that we recommend are *Homeopathic Medicine for Children and Infants* by Dana Ullman, M.P.H., and *The New Concise Guide to Homeopathy* by Nigel and Susan Garion-Hutchings.

Homeopathic remedies can be kept in your medicine cabinet alongside your first aid kit. They have an indefinite shelf life when handled and stored properly. Keep these medicines away from heat and sunlight and potent odors, such as perfumes. Though they taste sweet, they are medicines, so be sure to store them (and all medications) where children cannot reach them.

Homeopathic remedies are usually found in tablet or pellet form. You take them by letting them melt under the tongue. The remedies are most effective when you do not have anything to eat or drink for 15 minutes before and after you take them. They come in various strengths, although most homeopathic doctors agree that if you have the right remedy, the potency is not too important. The most common strengths are 12x and 9c (these are similar strengths), and the dose is usually 4 pellets for adults or 2 pellets for children, taken three times a day for five days, and as necessary after that. Be sure to read the directions and dosage on the bottle of homeopathic remedies that you purchase.

The following are some common homeopathic remedies that are used time and time again. You may want to keep them on hand.

- **Arsenicum**
- **Chamomilla**
- **Ignatia**
- **Nux vomica**
- **Pulsatilla**

→ MEDITATION ←

Guidelines for Meditation Practice

Generally, meditation has been associated with religious doctrines and disciplines as a means of becoming one with God or the universe, finding enlightenment, achieving selflessness, and other virtues. It is, however, a well-known fact that meditation can be practiced independently of any religious or philosophical orientation, purely as a means of reducing inner discord and increasing self-knowledge.

Meditation is an individual experience, but when people meditate together, the room is filled with wonderful energy that enhances the process. A weekly family meditation can be a great way to spend time together. This is also a great way to teach your children the importance of reflection. Our children can sit still for a fifteen-minute meditation. This is a good length of time to start with, and you can build it up as they get older. Adults should plan on 20 to 30 minutes for an effective meditation time.

The following guidelines will enable you to experience the benefits of meditation. If you remember that meditation, like sleep, does not need to be taught but comes naturally if you follow the right steps, you will progress rapidly and easily on your path.

1. Set aside a special place for meditation. It should be quiet and free of distractions. You should meditate in the same place each day if possible, because you create an atmosphere in your special place that will be conducive to further practice. Meditating in their bedrooms is especially beneficial for children. Doing so will create an atmosphere of peace in the room where they need to get good sleep and will build positive vibrations there.

2. Make sure that you are warm enough by choosing loose-fitting, comfortable clothing.

3. Meditate at the same time each day: this is essential for building a habit of meditation in your life. The morning and evening hours are good times to choose for your practice.

4. Instruct your mind to remain quiet for the duration of your meditation. If thoughts persist, just watch them come and go without involvement of any kind.

5. Plan your meditation with your eating needs in mind. Generally it is best to wait at least an hour after a meal. As meditation becomes a regular habit, you will begin to prefer to eat lightly before or after your practice.

6. Regulate the flow of your breath when you begin your meditation. It is helpful initially to focus on your breath and to breathe slowly and easily. This practice also aids you in controlling your mind. As you meditate, you should establish a slow, rhythmic breathing pattern that will allow your mind and body to relax in the meditation. Soon it will seem as if the breathing continues on its own without your conscious awareness of a need for control.

7. The more commonly used meditation postures are sitting and kneeling. It is helpful to sit or kneel on a pillow for added comfort and support. If sitting upright is uncomfortable for you, you can also meditate lying down. Whatever posture you select, you should maintain it with your back, neck, and head in a straight line, preferably facing the earth's magnetic poles to the north or east. When you meditate, you should feel steady and relaxed.

8. The traditional hand position is to rest your hands on your thighs with the tips of the thumb and index finger of each hand joined in the yogic chin mudra (finger position). This aids your meditation by allowing the energy in the meridians to flow freely to the fingertips and back up both your arms. If you find the position distracting, you also can meditate with your hands resting comfortably in an open position on your thighs.

Meditation Techniques

Because people have many different temperaments, many different meditative techniques have been developed. If you have never meditated, you might wish to try several of the following techniques to discover which one is the best for you. If your children respond to music, you can try playing an instrumental meditation tape. If your children are visual learners, you might start with *Tratak,* or "gazing" (see page 40). In any case, help your children get into the habit of meditating by setting aside quiet time for them each day.

Meditation is a time to let go of your daily tensions and anxieties, a time to let your mind and body relax and just be. It is also a time to gain insights into your inner resources.

Witnessing Witnessing is the purest form of meditation. It is simply sitting in meditation and watching the thoughts that come and go, without judging or commenting. It is interesting to see what our moment-to-moment thoughts consist of from a completely neutral position.

Vipassana *Vipassana* is a Buddhist meditation that focuses on the rise and fall of the breath. *Vipassana* means "breath." While the mind is engaged in focusing on your breathing, it cannot focus on its usual distractions. In this meditation, your breathing should be gentle and regular. Just allow it to be the place where your mind is focused and enjoy the feeling of witnessing breathing rather than concentrating on it.

Zazen *Zazen* means "just sitting." It is the basic meditation of Zen Buddhists, for whom the path of enlightenment is everyday life lived with awareness and totality. Like all meditations, Zazen is a tool to help us rediscover the immediacy and freshness of ordinary life, as we did as children. In Zazen, you just sit and allow whatever happens to happen. Your mind will try to distract you with past and present concerns to take you away from fully experiencing the moment. Zen Buddhists believe these transient thoughts are "paper tigers" and that paying attention to them only gives them more energy. In Zazen, you will experience the feeling of sitting and the fact that you are not the mind and can ignore its chatter at will. If your mind is particularly rebellious, you can give it a distraction to play with, such as concentrating on the breath.

Tratak (Gazing) Another device to still the mind so that you can experience directly is *Tratak,* or "gazing." The object that you look at is not really important. Traditional objects include a lighted candle, a flower, a religious image, or a picture of a guru. The main point of the exercise is to keep your eyes on a central spot because not moving the eyes restricts the input of information for your brain to process. The idea is to keep your mind quiet by keeping your thoughts simple. When you start to think about something else, keep bringing your attention back to the object of your contemplation. The goal of your meditation is to feel the quality of the object, to relax, and to enjoy what you are seeing.

Listening Meditation is centered on the idea of relaxing and nondoing. When you are thinking, you may hear but you cannot truly listen. Choose some music, chanting, or focus on natural sounds. Listen carefully and experience the essence of the sound, giving yourself the experience of emptiness, clarity, and receptivity.

Mantra In mantra meditation, you produce the sounds out loud or to yourself; either way, the sounds will produce an internal effect. In the Sanskrit language, *man* is translated as "mind" and *tra* means "protection." The repetition of the mantra or sound evokes a deep and peaceful reaction throughout your body.

Mantras are energies that are thought to have always existed in the universe. They pass in succession from teacher to disciple in an unbroken chain. The mantra leads the way to meditation and to a state of nonduality. Two typical Eastern mantras are "Om" (I am) and "So-Ham" (I am That).

A mantra can be anything that you enjoy repeating. The words "flower" or "one" are often used, as are names of saints or great teachers. For example, "Om Namah Shivaya" means "the God within." It should be repeated slowly, sounding each syllable: Om/Na/Mah/Shi/Va/Ya. Another, and perhaps the most widely used mantra in the world today, is "Om Mani Padme Hum." In Sanskrit *Om* represents the universal energy or life force; *Mani* means "jewel" or "crystal." *Padme* means "lotus," and *Hum* means "heart."

Ram Dass, in *The Only Dance There Is,* explains this mantra's meaning as follows: "The entire universe is like a pure jewel or crystal within the heart of the lotus flower, which represents myself, and it is manifest in my own heart."

Choose a mantra that feels right to you. You can chant it out loud or repeat it subvocally. Mantras are often used in conjunction with the Vipassana to bring about a deeper meditation.

Meditation in Action Everything can become a meditation, including the most ordinary everyday chores. What transforms daily activities into meditation action is awareness and wholeheartedness.

The application of the Zen exhortation to give undivided attention to and really feel the quality of each of your actions is exemplified in the Japanese tea ceremony and the art of flower arranging. Being present in the moment imparts an unmistakable peace, effortlessness, and enjoyment to the "little things" that make up the greater whole of life.

→ **YOGA** ←

Yogic postures, called *asanas*, help to stimulate the flow of energy in the body and stimulate the body's organs, which promotes wellness. They will enhance your energy and give you a feeling of well-being.

By practicing Yoga on a regular basis, you will develop skills and a limberness of body that will serve you well in any particular healing problem. When consistently practiced, Yoga is beneficial for health. When you practice specific yogic postures regularly, it will be easy for you to use them when the need arises. Yoga must be practiced for a period of time to develop the technique and the stamina and also to relax while in the postures.

The practice of Yoga is beneficial to children as well as to adults. Parents who teach Yoga to their children help them learn to relax and to balance their bodies. Parents benefit at the same time.

When practicing Yoga, find an area of your house that is quiet and well ventilated. You also need to have enough space to move freely. *If you have any physical problems, consult your physician before you attempt any Yoga poses.* Some other things to consider are:

- → Do not practice Yoga on a full stomach.
- → Do not practice Yoga when you are extremely fatigued.
- → Wear loose-fitting, comfortable clothing.
- → Practice on a clean mat or towel.
- → The room should be warm enough to exercise comfortably.
- → Turn off the television or radio. However, soft music playing in the background is beneficial.
- → Empty your bladder before starting.
- → Hold poses for an equal amount of time on each side of your body.
- → Have a "cool down" after stretching.
- → Proper breathing techniques make any yogic posture more effective.
- → If practicing Yoga with a child, work only as long as your child is enjoying it: no more than 45 minutes at a time.

The following three poses are excellent for general health. They encourage proper breathing techniques and keep the spine flexible, which allows the free flow of energy throughout the body. We like to start the day each morning with this practice.

THE COMPLETE BREATH

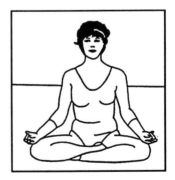

Basic position:
You may stand, sit, or lie on your back to do the exercise. Focus on a steady and continuous flow of air from the lowest to the highest portion of your lungs. Breathe continuously and as slowly as possible.

Instructions:

→ Inhale and fill the lower part of your lungs (your abdomen should expand gently). Continue inhaling and fill the upper portion of your lungs by expanding the upper part of your chest (your chest will rise slowly).

→ To fill the uppermost part of your lungs, slightly draw in your lower abdomen.

→ At the end of your inhalation, occasionally raise your shoulders to permit the air to enter the upper lobes of your lungs.

→ Retain your breath for as long as you comfortably can.

→ Exhale slowly and contract your abdomen slightly.

→ When the air is completely exhaled, relax your chest and abdomen.

Practice this exercise frequently, and do it whenever you become tense and tired. Do your inhalations and exhalations very slowly to allow ample time to complete each step. After just a few days of practice you will begin to find that the Complete Breath revitalizes and cleanses your body and brings about a deep sense of peace.

Benefits:

The Complete Breath is an exercise that can be practiced before or after any other yogic posture or routine. This exercise increases your lung capacity. It helps to cleanse your blood and expands your chest cavity, allowing all parts of your lungs to be filled with oxygen.

THE PLOW

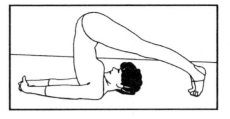

Basic position:
Lie flat on your back with your arms
at your sides.

Instructions:

→ Bring your knees up to your ears and support your back with your
  hands.
→ Gently extend your legs back until your toes touch the floor.
→ Keep your legs as straight as possible without straining and, if you wish,
  bring your hands gently down to the floor behind your back.
→ Hold the position for as long as it is comfortable.
→ Slowly return to the basic position, using your hands to support your
  back.
→ In the beginning, if you feel unsteady in the Plow, keep your hands on
  your back until you have gained more flexibility and confidence.
→ Repeat four times.

Breathing:
Inhale deeply and exhale fully before starting.
Keep your lungs empty while rolling back.
Breathe normally in the final position.
Keep your lungs empty as you return to the basic position.

Limitations:
Do not practice the asana if you have sciatica or lower back pain, or are
menstruating heavily.

Benefits:

Stretches the spine; tones the kidneys, liver, and gallbladder; limbers the pelvis and legs; and improves digestion.

THE FISH

Basic position:

Lie flat on the floor with your arms at your sides.

Instructions:

- → Arch your back.
- → Slide your hands under your buttocks.
- → Tilt your head back until the top of your head rests on the floor.
- → Remain in the posture as long as you comfortably can.
- → Slowly return to the basic position.
- → Repeat four or five times.

Breathing:

Breathe deeply and slowly in the posture.

Benefits:

Strengthens the abdominal muscles; helps recirculate stagnant blood; and aids in regulating the thyroid gland.

3

Building a Healthy Lifestyle

Having a healthy life is a matter of leading a healthy lifestyle. That means taking care of yourself: body, mind, and spirit. If parents and children are individually healthy, then together they create a healthy family and a healthy lifestyle in general. In this chapter we'll discuss building a healthy way of life—both mentally and physically—for your family. At the end of the chapter, you'll find suggestions for daily activities and routines that will strengthen you and those you love and that will help prevent your family from becoming ill.

⤙ BODY ⤚

A good diet is essential for the body. In the Eastern traditions, the human body is considered to be a microcosm of the universe requiring a balance of yin and yang energy to function properly. Therefore, it is thought that the most nutritious diet consists of simple foods that are balanced and in harmony with their natural sources. An individual's body, his or her food, and the immediate surroundings are seen as three interrelated energy forms. The energy that food imparts is related not only to its taste and flavor but to the way it is prepared, the quality of its selection, the way it is cut, the length of cooking time, the amount of seasoning, and how the meal is presented.

Cooking is considered a very important function in an Eastern household because the cook is responsible for the health and wellbeing of the family. If the person who prepares the family's food cooks with consideration and care, the members of the family are filled with energy and vibrant health. He or she also provides an atmosphere that is conducive to enjoyment of the meal. Ideally, there is always a harmonious balance of colors at the table as well as a variety of tastes. Foods are never served too hot or too cold, too spicy or too bland. Seasonal changes are also taken into consideration; freshly grown produce is preferable to food that has been packaged or processed.

If it is at all possible, a healthy family lifestyle would include the family's sitting down to eat together at least once or twice a week. This allows the family members to interact and learn to enjoy one another and share their individual experiences.

Quality breathing is an important part of staying healthy. Every one of our cells is affected by the quality of our breath. Just as when we are active, we become hungry; when we are active, the cells in our body need extra oxygen. The more work they do, the more oxygen they need. Every time cells work, oxidation takes place and energy is created. The end product, or residue, of oxidation is the waste product carbon dioxide. This process is similar to fuel burning and leaving a residue of ashes. Just as a fire cannot burn without oxygen for combustion, our cells cannot burn their nutrients without oxidation. When we breathe, stored energy is activated within each of our cells. Our bodies are then able to move and remain warm because one-third of the energy produced is used for action while the other two-thirds becomes heat energy.

Both parents and children can improve the quality of their breathing by incorporating more exercise in their lifestyle. Children should play more outside instead of sitting in front of the TV, and adults should play sports or play with their children. Family outings are also a wonderful way to move the body and create a greater energy flow. Smoking limits a person's ability to take in a full breath, so you should stop smoking, for your health and the health of your whole family. There are many organizations available to help you quit. Ask your doctor or check with your local hospital for resources in your area.

Exercise is important for keeping our bodies healthy. Some kinds of exercise are especially helpful in promoting energy and vitality. Walking, for example, is a natural exercise for humans. The only thing needed is a good, comfortable pair of shoes. The risk of injury is minimal, and you can walk just about anywhere and anytime. A family walk after dinner helps you to digest and gives you time together to talk.

Families can do many forms of exercise together, such as bicycle riding, hiking, swimming, and dancing.

The world contains many forms of toxins. Some toxins to avoid include:

> **All kinds of stress**
> **Chemical additives in processed foods**
> **Polyunsaturated fats and hydrogenated oils**
> **Alcoholic beverages**
> **Caffeine, coffee**
> **Tobacco smoke**
> **Pollution**

It is important to minimize your exposure to toxins wherever possible.

Since our bodies are made up mostly of water, it is important that we all drink lots of pure water every day. There's no substitute for plain, pure water when it comes to keeping our bodies healthy. Parents should pack a bottle of plain water in their children's backpacks and encourage them to drink throughout their school day. Drinking water is the best way to help flush toxins out of the system.

Bodywork is another way of keeping in good health. It can be used for specific stress problems or other problems that you may have, and it can certainly improve anyone's sense of well-being. We highly recommend these therapies for both adults and children. Bodywork is therapeutic work done on the body, and it comes in a variety of styles. Here we discuss osteopathy, chiropractic, and massage, although there are other forms that you may find fit your lifestyle better.

The founder of osteopathy, Andrew Taylor Still, was a physician on the Union side during the American Civil War. He became disillusioned with the orthodox medical practices of the time and started treating his patients with his system for adjusting the spine. The spinal cord regulates the functioning of the autonomic nervous system, and the spine also sends messages to the muscles and skeletal system. Osteopaths believe that keeping these two systems balanced and aligned is of prime importance in a patient's health care.

If you or your child seems to be developing physical symptoms, such as headaches or back pain, it may be an indication that the body is not balanced and aligned. A visit to an osteopathic physician may prove beneficial. Today most osteopaths are family practitioners, and their degree is D.O., or doctor of osteopathy.

Chiropractic was founded in 1895 by David D. Palmer of Iowa. He believed that a displacement in any part of the skeletal frame would cause nerve dysfunction. Therefore, chiropractic is based on the idea that the spinal column is central to one's entire sense of well-being, as it is instrumental in maintaining the health of the nervous system. Another vital chiropractic concept is that if the body is functioning in a balanced way, it can cure its own illnesses and keep itself in perfect health.

Slight displacements of the spinal vertebrae, called subluxations, can be reflected in a wide range of symptoms. The aim of the chiropractor, therefore, is to find the subluxation and correct it manually.

Massage has been effective in raising energy levels and reducing stress and tension. It improves the circulation in the muscles and tissues and stimulates circulation in the deeper blood vessels and lymphatic system. During massage, toxic waste material is carried away from the cells. Immediate effects can be observed in the rosy color of the skin.

⇥ MIND ⇤

Taking care of your mind can be challenging and wonderful for you and your child. Make sure that you are stimulated by your work and that you enjoy what you are doing. You and other family members can read inspirational books. Learn new things. Engage in lively conversation. Play word games; write in a journal. Avoid negative thoughts, especially before bed. Always try to get a good night's sleep.

Bedtime is an ideal time to spend with your child getting ready for a good night's sleep. Parents can read books to their children, play special music, or just talk. This is a positive habit to get into and one that will create long-lasting memories for all of you.

⇥ SPIRIT ⇤

To take care of your spirit, do things that make you feel happy. Stop and smell the roses! Keep flowers in your home. Spend time with friends. Give yourself time alone. Spend time in silence. Spend time in nature. Pray, meditate, chant, or do whatever you like to do to keep in touch with your Higher Power.

Music can be used to create an extremely beneficial deep state of relaxation. Music allows you to move into another dimension, where you can become completely aware of the sounds that you hear. This state can release the stresses and tensions that you are carrying. The act of listening to soothing music allows your muscles to relax, your mind to become peaceful, and all of the organs in your body to function more slowly, thereby allowing your entire system to enter a deep state of rest. Since each person responds differently to music, it is important to select music that is peaceful and soothing to you. When you listen to music for the purpose of relaxation, you should set aside at least 15 minutes of uninterrupted time.

→ ACUPRESSURE ←

For thousands of years, acupressure has been used to bring about and maintain mind/body harmony. Acupressure is an extremely powerful method because it balances the body's entire energy system. It is like having all of the roads and freeways of the body running smoothly. Following a general routine of pressing the following acupressure points will help you and your child keep all of the body's energy flow balanced. The following points also will help to guide you into the quietness necessary to have a quality meditation. They represent a simple but very effective routine that can be done easily in 12 minutes each morning. You and your child or spouse will start your day off feeling revitalized and centered.

Press these points on both sides of the body for about 2 minutes each. You and your child can press these points daily, or at least three times a week.

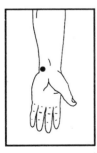

1ST WRIST POINT
(Heart 7)

On the inside crease of the wrist, and the little finger side of the hand.

Benefits:
Useful for insomnia, nervousness, sleepiness.

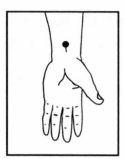

2ND WRIST POINT
(Pericardium 6)

On the inside of the arm, about 2 inches up from the crease of the wrist, between the two large bones of the forearm. *Do not use on pregnant women.*

Benefits:

Useful for relieving depression, dizziness, nausea, nervousness, sleepiness.

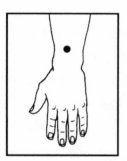

BACK OF WRIST POINT
(Triple Warmer 5)

About 2 inches up from the back of the wrist, between the two bones of the forearm.

Benefits:

Useful for relieving hypertension, depression, headache, or nervousness.

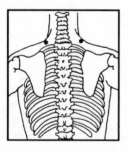

SHOULDER POINT
(Gallbladder 21)

Where the shoulder meets the neck, on the line where the back meets the front.

Benefits:

Useful for neck and shoulder tension, nervousness.

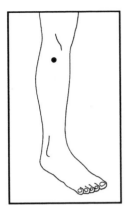

LEG POINT
(Stomach 36)

About 3 inches below the kneecap, just off the edge of the shin. *Do not use on pregnant women.*

Benefits:
Useful for fatigue, headache, nausea, nervousness, stomach upset.

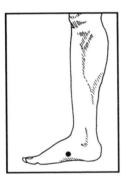

ARCH POINT
(Spleen 4)

Located in the arch of the inside foot, slightly be-hind the center of the arch. *Do not use on pregnant women.*

Benefits:
Useful for nervousness.

⇥ AROMATHERAPY ⇤

It is easy and fun to make aromatherapy part of your life. In the morning, to help wake you up and lift your spirit, scent the kitchen with a spicy-citrusy blend like orange-cinnamon. You can place some orange peel and cinnamon sticks in water and let them boil awhile on the stove while you're fixing breakfast.

You can carry an aroma with you throughout the day, wearing it as a perfume or on a cotton ball tucked inside your desk. Breathe in your favorite aroma when you are feeling hassled or stressed. Basil and rosemary are good to have at the office. You can even keep live plants there and pick off the leaves as you need them!

After work, you can settle the atmosphere with some scented candles; rose or gardenia are especially nice.

Before bed, you can prepare for sleep with chamomile or lavender.

You can use any one of the tools given in Chapter 2 to enhance your child's room with a variety of aromas. Stimulating, citrusy aromas will help him or her wake up, and calming, floral aromas will help him or her to sleep.

When guests visit, it is refreshing to have potpourri set out in the bathrooms. Fresh, fragrant flowers are welcome in any room of the house.

⇒ AYURVEDA ⇐

Ayurveda is best used as a preventive medicine. Keeping your mind and body in balance is an ongoing commitment that will keep you healthy. The Ayurvedic lifestyle may seem cumbersome at first, but once you get into the routine and experience the benefits of increased energy and vitality, you'll love it!

Your mind/body type, discussed in Chapter 2, will determine what kinds of foods you should favor and what kinds of exercise you should do. But regardless of mind/body type, there are certain things that everyone can do on a daily basis to benefit from Ayurveda. You can choose to do as much or as little as is comfortable for your lifestyle. The longer you practice Ayurveda, the easier it becomes, until it is second nature.

Ayurveda recommends reading the *Bhagavad Gita* for spiritual nourishment. From this text, a set of behavior *rasayanas,* or behavioral recommendations, has been developed. It is said that following these instructions will help you avoid contradictions in the mind and, therefore, prevent symptoms caused by that strain.

Behavior Rayasanas

→ Be truthful, speak sweetly.

→ Be free from anger.

→ Abstain from immoderate behavior.

→ Be nonviolent and calm.

→ Observe cleanliness in yourself and your environment.

→ Be charitable toward others.

→ Observe a regular daily routine.

→ Be loving and compassionate.

→ Be respectful to teachers and elders.

→ Keep the company of the wise.

→ Be unconceited, well mannered, and simple in behavior.

→ Follow your religious beliefs, be self-controlled.

→ Keep a positive outlook.

→ Devote yourself to the development of higher states of consciousness.

It is not necessary to memorize these rasayanas, as doing so may put strain on the mind. Just read them every day to remind yourself of the simple things you can do to help yourself and, in turn, to help the world.

Here's what you'll need to get started with an Ayurvedic routine:

→ sesame oil (cured, light, for Ayurvedic massage)

You also may want to obtain these tools to use in your routine:

→ a tongue scraper
→ ambrosia and nectar (Ayurvedic "vitamins")
→ Ayurvedic tea (in Vata, Pitta, and/or Kapha)
→ a copper cup
→ churnas (Ayurvedic spices designed to balance the three doshas) to sprinkle on food

These things and more can be ordered from the Healing Arts Center or from the Maharishi Ayur-Ved Products catalog. (See Appendix 2.)

Ideal Daily Ayurvedic Routine
→ Wake up at sunrise, about 6:00 A.M.
→ Drink water that's been left in the copper cup overnight. (This helps prepare the body for elimination of waste.)
→ Use the bathroom, emptying your bowels and bladder.
→ Brush your teeth, then clean your tongue with the tongue scraper to promote oral health and hygiene.
→ Give yourself an Ayurvedic massage. (Instructions are on page 28.)
→ Do your Yoga (Sun Salutations are recommended in this chapter) and/or your exercise program.
→ Take a warm shower or bath.
→ Meditate. Ayurveda recommends transcendental meditation. (See Chapter 2 for more information.)

→ Eat a light breakfast based on your mind/body type diet.

→ Take your Ayurvedic herbs or "vitamins" for increased vitality.

→ Work or study.

→ Eat lunch, your largest meal of the day, at the same time each day, between noon and 1:00 P.M.

→ Work or study.

→ Meditate before dinner.

→ Eat a light dinner, at the same time each day, preferably before 6:30 P.M.

→ Take your Ayurvedic herbs.

→ Take a short walk to aid digestion.

→ Relax. Read. Listen to music. Visit with friends.

→ Get to bed by 10:00 P.M.

Of course, you may adapt the routine to accommodate your schedule. For example, if your mornings are hectic and you need to leave the house very early, you may choose to do your massage and shower in the evening. Doing so will give you an especially restful night's sleep. If you wake up hungry, as many of us do, you may choose to eat breakfast before your shower. Ayurveda will prove beneficial in whatever way it is blended into your routine. Even just adding a couple of new things into your established routine will give you a good start.

Here are a few ideas that will help you to incorporate the Ayurvedic routine into your family's lifestyle:

→ Parents can drink Ayurvedic tea with their breakfast.

→ Spices for specific mind/body types can be sprinkled onto food easily with *churnas,* which are packaged herbs in shaker jars that can be left on the table. These herbs promote strong digestion, which Ayurveda teaches is essential for good health.

→ Parents can massage infants and young children with sesame oil before their baths.

→ A morning family walk on the weekends starts the day off right.

The most important part of the Ayurvedic routine is meditation, which is discussed in detail in Chapter 2.

It is nice to take your time in the morning and fit in all of the Ayurvedic routine, but if you are in a hurry, it is better to do it all quickly rather than to skip it altogether.

You can have your tea with meals, during an afternoon break, or after dinner. You can sprinkle the churnas on any foods to give you the tastes recommended to balance the doshas.

→ BACH FLOWERS ←

If you want to carry a single Bach Flower remedy with you, the one to choose is Rescue Remedy. This remedy is a combination of five different Bach Flowers: Cherry Plum, Clematis, Impatiens, Rock Rose, and Star of Bethlehem. It is an all-purpose remedy for all kinds of emergencies. It helps relieve trauma, anguish, or even daily stress buildup. It is also useful when you have anxiety about an upcoming test or a trip to the dentist. This convenient Bach Flower remedy can be administered to adults and children for a variety of purposes.

⇀ COLOR THERAPY ↼

You are being influenced by color every day, whether you realize it or not. Restaurants and businesses plan their decor with the customers' reaction to color in mind. Be aware of the impact of colors and use them to create the atmosphere you desire.

Cool colors—blues and greens—are soothing and calming. These colors are wonderful in the bedroom or any place you want to relax.

Warm colors—reds, oranges, and yellows—are stimulating. These colors work well in the kitchen and family room, where you want to stimulate appetites and make people feel warm and welcome.

The classic navy blue "interview" suit came about because it looks crisp and professional. A warm-colored tie or scarf warms up the outfit and makes you more approachable and friendly.

White is known to be cooling while in the sun because it reflects light. It also reflects energy and will protect you from negativity. Black, on the other hand, absorbs light and energy from whatever source it picks up on. Black and other dark colors give weight and a sense of stability to a room.

⇀ HERBS ↼

The easiest way to add herbs to your daily routine is by including them in your diet. Three roots, if eaten regularly, will help to keep you healthy; they are garlic, ginger, and onion.

All of these are found in just about any supermarket and can ward off health problems before they start.

→ **Peppermint tea** is a stimulating beverage that can take the place of coffee to get you going in the morning. It is also a delicious drink for kids to help them wake up and be alert for school. It can be served iced in the summer for a refreshing treat.

→ **Ginger tea** is nice to have after lunch to help you digest.

→ **Chamomile tea** is wonderful after dinner when you want to settle down and relax.

→ MEDITATION ←

Daily meditation is a very important part of developing and maintaining a healthy lifestyle. For most people, meditation is most effective if done first thing in the morning, before the hustle and bustle of daily activity begins. This is the time when the mind is quietest and most receptive to the benefits of meditation. Another very important time to meditate is just before going to bed. Meditation at this time quiets the mind and relaxes the body, which prepares you for restful and health-producing sleep. A daily routine of meditation, that would include 20 minutes in the morning and 20 minutes in the evening is ideal. You may need to establish the meditation practice with a child by sitting with him or her and encouraging him or her to relax and focus. This is a habit that will bring lifelong benefits, including an increase in overall energy level and clarity of thought.

Aromatherapy is a useful tool in helping to prepare the atmosphere for meditation. It also can calm the mind and get the body in a more relaxed state so that it can be recharged. Many people like to burn incense or scented candles during meditation.

Choose a fragrance that appeals to you. These scents in particular have been known to enhance meditation:

- **Clary-sage**
- **Geranium**
- **Jonquil**
- **Patchouli**

Guided meditation tapes are another good tool for meditation. There are many different tapes available. You can check the New Age section of your local record store or order from the Healing Arts Center. Music that quiets the mind and brings tranquillity to the environment is also extremely helpful to a quality meditation.

Here's an easy meditation that all family members can use to get started:

Healthy Family Meditation

- Find a quiet place where you will not be disturbed and turn on some soft music.
- Sit in a comfortable position so that your back is as straight as it can be without feeling stiff.
- Place your hands on your lap and put your feet flat on the floor.
- Close your eyes.
- Begin breathing rhythmically and deeply. Bring your mind to focus completely on your breath.
- On the in-breath, repeat to yourself, "I am." On the out-breath, repeat to yourself, "Relaxed." Continue this for 2 to 3 minutes.
- Then envision your body encapsulated in a beautiful cocoon of

blue light. Allow your body to relax in this blue cocoon for 5 minutes.

→ Become aware of your breath once again and repeat on the in-breath, "I am" and on the out-breath, "refreshed and revitalized." Continue this process for 2 to 3 minutes.

This simple routine takes only about 10 minutes, but it will greatly enhance your whole day or your night's sleep by bringing your body into balance. For variety or to fulfill special needs, you can add any of the other meditation techniques discussed in various chapters or styles of meditation included in Chapter 2. However, this very easy routine is extremely beneficial for everyone in the family, from the oldest member to young children.

→ YOGA ←

Once you have released the tension in your body and balanced your energy, building a healthy lifestyle is much easier. Yoga is excellent for letting go of frustration and those feelings of heaviness that keep us from moving forward. People who do a series of Yoga postures at least three times a week find that the entire week goes more smoothly.

Because kids love to do Yoga, it's a fun way to spend time together. The fact that a lot of poses are named after animals allows them to use their imagination and makes exercise fun. When parents do Yoga with children, parent–child relations are improved. Teaching your child Yoga helps him or her learn to relax and to balance his or her body. In the meantime, it will help you also.

The following daily Yoga routine promotes general good health and flexibility as well as a sense of well-being. A daily practice of the Sun Salutation keeps the body and mind in perfect harmony. It is the morning routine practiced around the world and considered by Yoga enthusiasts to be the essential combination of poses to keep the mind still and the body balanced.

Help your child learn the routine. One set takes about 3 to 4 minutes. After you and your child have perfected the moves, do at least three sets per session. Louise uses this routine to start her day each morning.

Sun Salutation

The twelve positions of this exercise should be done slowly and rhythmically.

POSITION I. PRAYER POSE

(*Pranamasana*)

Exhale. Stand straight. Place your palms together in front of your chest.
Relax your body.

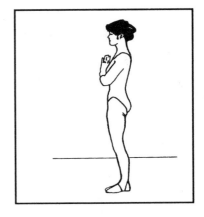

POSITION 2. RAISED-ARMS POSE
(*Hasta Uttanasana*)

Inhale. Stretch your arms above your head, keeping them shoulder-width apart. Bend backward as far as you can.

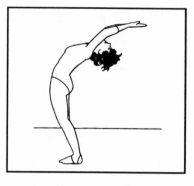

POSITION 3. HAND-TO-FOOT POSE
(*Padahastasana*)

Exhale. Stretch forward until your hands touch the floor next to your feet. Bring your forehead close to your knees and keep your legs as straight as possible.

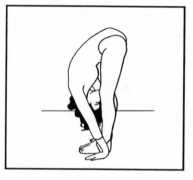

POSITION 4. EQUESTRIAN POSE
(*Ashwa Sanchalanasana*)

Inhale. With a backward step, stretch your right leg away from your body with your knee touching the floor. Keep the palms of your hands beside your left foot. Arch your back and look up.

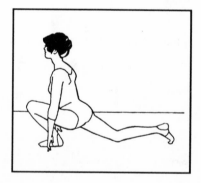

POSITION 5. QUADRUPED POSE

(Catuspadasana)

Exhale. Hold your breath out, and move your left leg back so that you are resting on your hands and toes in a push-up position. Keep your back and head straight.

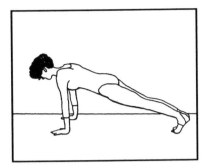

POSITION 6. SALUTE WITH EIGHT LIMBS

(Ashtanga Namaskara)

Inhale. As you exhale, lower your body to the floor keeping your hips and abdomen raised. Your toes, knees, and chest should touch the floor.

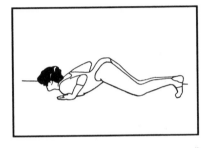

POSITION 7. THE SERPENT POSE

(Bhujangasna)

Inhale. Straighten your arms as you raise your upper body from the waist. Bend backward as far as you can, looking up and back.

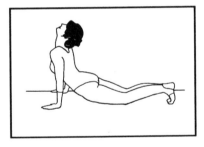

POSITION 8. THE MOUNTAIN POSE

(Parvatasana)

Exhale. Put your heels down so that your feet are flat on the floor. Lift your body up to form a triangle. Keep your head down and your arms and legs straight.

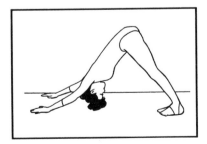

POSITION 9. EQUESTRIAN POSE
(*Ashwa Sanvhalanasana*)

Inhale. Bring your right foot
forward next to your hands and,
at the same time, lower your left
knee to the floor.
Arch your back and look up.

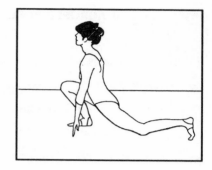

POSITION 10. HAND-TO-FOOT POSE
(*Padahastasana*)

Exhale. Stretch forward until
your hands are in line with your
feet. Bring your forehead close to
your knees and keep your legs
as straight as possible.

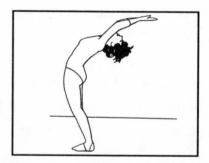

POSITION 11. RAISED-ARMS POSE
(*Hasta Uttanasana*)

Inhale. Stretch your arms over your
head. Bend as far backward as you
comfortably can.

POSITION 12. PRAYER POSE
(*Pranamasana*)

Exhale. Stand straight.
Place your palms together
in front of your chest.
Relax your body.

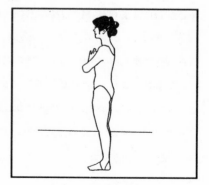

You may want to do the following additional poses at the end of the Sun Salutation. All these poses help to balance the body, stimulate the mind, and calm the spirit. They can be done alternately or they can form a routine all their own. If you choose to add these to your routine, be sure to perform them after you conclude the Sun Salutation. These poses are a little more difficult, and the Sun Salutation will warm up your body for these advanced moves.

KING OF DANCER'S POSE

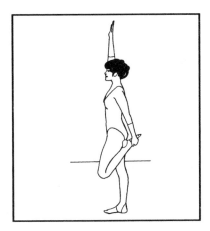

Basic position:
Stand with your feet shoulder-width apart. Be sure your weight is distributed evenly and your arms are relaxed at your sides.

Instructions:
→ Focus your eyes on a specific point in front of you while keeping your head straight.
→ Raise your left foot and reach back with your left hand to grasp your foot firmly.
→ Raise your right arm. Try to maintain your balance.
→ Continue stretching upward as you hold the position.
→ Hold the position as long as you wish.
→ Slowly return to the original position.
→ Change legs and repeat.
→ Do the asana three times on each side.

Breathing:

Inhale while bringing your arm and leg together.

Breathe normally while in the posture.

Inhale while returning to the starting position.

Limitations:

If you have a weak stomach or back muscles, you should not attempt this exercise until you first strengthen these muscles with other asanas.

Benefits:

Balances the nervous system; promotes bodily control and mental concentration; strengthens the back, legs, and hips.

FOOT-BALANCING POSE

Basic Position:

Stand with your feet approximately 4 to 6 inches apart. Distribute the weight of your body evenly on both feet, arms comfortably at your sides.

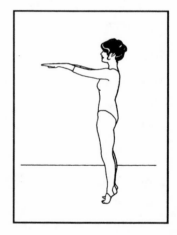

Instructions:

→ Gently lift your arms in front of you; your elbows may be slightly bent for balance. Simultaneously, rise up onto your toes.

→ Hold the asana as long as you comfortably can.

→ Slowly return to your original position.

→ Repeat between five and ten times.

Breathing:

Inhale as you raise your heels and stretch out your arms. Breathe normally in the asana. Exhale as you lower your heels and your arms.

Benefits:

Strengthens the back, stomach, legs, and feet and helps to develop balance and correct posture.

THE TRIANGLE POSE

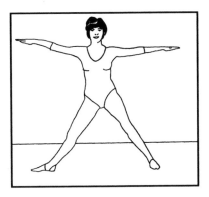

Basic Position:

Stand with your legs wide apart. Turn your right foot out approximately 90 degrees and your left foot in approximately 30 degrees. Be sure that the heel of your right foot is directly in line with the middle of your left foot. Raise your arms to shoulder level.

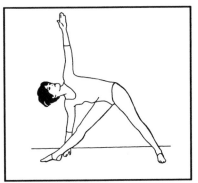

Instructions:

→ Bend from the hip slowly to the right side, keeping both of your hips in an even line.

→ Bring your right hand to your ankle or calf, or where you can reach without straining.

→ Extend your left arm vertically and, if you wish, look up at your hand. Do not be discouraged if at first you do not reach the completed stretch.

→ Slowly return to the basic position.

→ Repeat on the other side. (Be sure to change the foot position.) Repeat three times on each side.

Breathing:

Inhale while raising your arms. Exhale while bending to the side. Hold your breath out while stretching.

Benefits:

Stimulates the nervous system, improves digestion, gently massages the spinal nerves and muscles of the lower back and abdominal organs.

UPRIGHT HEAD-TO-KNEE POSE

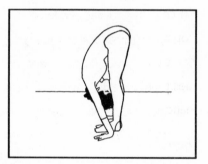

Basic Position:

Stand straight with your feet comfortably apart. Extend your arms straight in front of you.

Instructions:

→ Bend forward and place your hands next to your feet, or clasp your hands behind your legs.

→ Bring your head as close as possible into the space between your knees. Your legs should remain as straight as possible throughout the stretch.

→ Hold between 5 and 10 seconds.

→ Slowly return to your original position.

→ Repeat five times.

Breathing:

Inhale deeply and exhale fully before bending. Exhale while bending.
Breathe normally in the complete stretch. Inhale as you straighten up.

Benefits:

Stimulates the pancreas, relaxes the hamstring muscles and hip joints, massages the spinal nerves, and brings a rich blood supply to the brain.

SHOULDER ROTATIONS

Basic Position:

Sit cross-legged or in a half-lotus (the
top of one foot resting on your thigh,
the other foot on the floor tucked under the other thigh) position with your
hands on your knees.

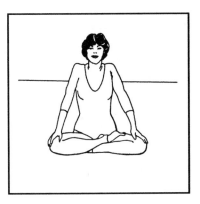

Instructions:

- ✦ Slowly rotate your shoulders forward in a large circle.
- ✦ Repeat five times.
- ✦ Change direction and repeat five more times.

Breathing:

Inhale slowly while raising your shoulders.
Exhale slowly as your shoulders come down.

Benefits:

Loosens the shoulder joints and relieves tension in the shoulders and
upper back.

A HEALTHY MORNING ROUTINE

+ Arise at sunrise

+ Meditate for 10 to 20 minutes

+ Sesame oil massage (see page 28)

+ Yoga routine: Sun Salutation

+ Shower

+ Eat a light breakfast based on your Ayurvedic mind/body type

A HEALTHY EVENING ROUTINE

+ Eat a light dinner no later than 6:30 P.M.

+ Take a short walk

+ Relax; listen to music

+ Do some Yoga postures according to your body's needs

+ Meditate for 10 to 20 minutes

+ Get to bed by 10:00 P.M.

This is an ideal daily routine for adults. You may adapt it to fit your daily schedule and to fit the needs of younger members of the household. Incorporating any portion of this routine into your life should prove beneficial. To accomplish your family's lifestyle goals, you may add other remedies discussed elsewhere in this book.

4

Colds and Flus and the Stuff That Goes with Them

The common cold is called "common" because it happens so frequently and to so many of us. No matter what time of year it is, anyone can come down with a cold.

A runny nose and watery eyes may be the first indication that your child is coming down with a cold. It is good to catch the symptoms at this stage to avoid further complications such as sore throat, coughing, tiredness, and achy muscles. Your child may also develop a mild fever. If the fever persists or begins to rise, consult your doctor. A fever may indicate an infection and needs to be diagnosed by a physician.

Colds are contagious, so when you've got one, avoid contact with other people, including other family members. Every family member should wash his or her hands frequently to help keep the germs from spreading. While there is no cure for this annoying little disease, there are plenty of ways to minimize the symptoms so you can feel better until the cold runs its course and goes away.

A flu can range from a really bad cold to a near-death experience.

It is caused by a virus, whereas some colds may be caused by bacteria. Most of the time, the difference between a cold and the flu is that the flu also affects the stomach.

The old "chicken soup" remedy is actually a good idea because the soup has some excellent medicinal qualities. The steam from the soup helps to clear the sinuses, and the vegetables contain vitamins that help boost your immune system. It's a good idea to increase your intake of clear fluids to help the body flush out toxins. Avoid milk—it will just cause your body to produce more mucus. Also avoid chocolate when you have a cold because chocolate can irritate the throat and can deplete a body of much-needed vitamin B.

Here are some other things you can do when you or someone you love has a cold or the flu.

→ ACUPRESSURE ←

Colds and flu often begin when we are tired or under emotional stress. When our resistance is low, our system is most receptive to colds and the flu virus. Acupressure is very effective in preventing colds and flu as well as in alleviating the symptoms. It can be used for low resistance, chills, runny nose, coughing, headache, sinus, sore throat, chest congestion, and low energy—all possible symptoms that accompany colds and flu.

Use the acupressure points that follow for 1 to 2 minutes each and repeat them three to four times daily. The points are easy for children to use on themselves, but the pressure should be firm and steady. As your child stimulates these points on him- or herself, do the same thing to yourself, so you won't catch the cold.

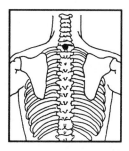

BACK OF NECK POINT
(Governing Vessel 14)

Located at the base of the back of the neck on the large knob in the middle.

Benefits:
Useful for colds, influenza, fever, stiff neck, vomiting, coughing.

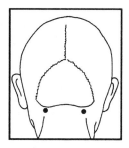

BASE OF SKULL POINT
(Gallbladder 20)

Located at the base of the skull in the hollowed-out depressions just behind the ears.

Benefits:
Useful for headaches, colds, influenza, fever, coughing, eye problems, stiff neck.

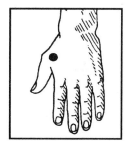

BACK OF HAND POINT
(Large Intestine 4)

Located on the fleshy muscle between the thumb and index finger bones. *Do not use on pregnant women.*

Benefits:
Useful for frontal headache, sinus trouble, colds, influenza, coughing, sore throat.

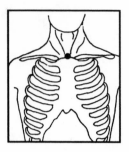

TOP OF STERNUM POINT

(Conception Vessel 22)

Located in the depression just at the base of the throat.

Benefits:
Useful for colds, coughs, chest congestion, sore throat, difficult breathing.

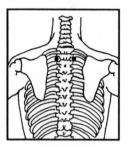

1ST UPPER BACK POINT

(Bladder 12)

Located next to the spine in line with the top of the scapula.

Benefits:
Useful for chest congestion, coughs, influenza, colds, breathing difficulties.

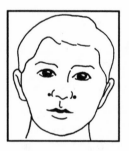

NOSTRIL POINT

(Large Intestine 20)

Located just beside the nostrils.

Benefits:
Useful for runny nose, sinus, nose cold, influenza, aching face, nosebleeds.

THIRD EYE POINT

(Yin-tang)

Located just between the eyebrows on the midline of the face.

Benefits:

Useful for headaches, sinus, runny nose, dizziness, sneezing, eye problems.

✦ AROMATHERAPY ✦

Any of the following oils can be used to help improve the symptoms of a cold or the flu:

✦ **Eucalyptus** can be used to treat many different cold symptoms. It is also helpful to those suffering from hay fever. It alleviates a cough, whether dry or with mucus, and can help to bring down a fever.

✦ **Lavender** and **Peppermint** both help with a fever and are particularly effective headache remedies. They also can reduce nausea.

✦ **Thyme** works on a cough and can be used in combination with eucalyptus.

✦ **Tea tree oil** is effective with all kinds of infections. It can be added to a thyme-eucalyptus blend to improve a cough with mucus.

✦ AYURVEDA ✦

It is important to know and understand your own mind/body type to correctly practice Ayurveda. When the body is in a state of balance, it is healthy. Use the remedy for your body type to put your body back into balance when you have a cold or the flu. Be familiar with the mind/body type of your child, too, so that you can help put his or her body back into balance when you need to.

The cold winter months, November through February, are the Vata season in Ayurveda. This is the time when Vata is more likely to become out of balance and result in a cold or the flu. Ayurveda traditionally recommends a routine for each season to maintain balance during that season. Of course, you should follow your own daily Ayurvedic plan, but make adjustments to fit with the season. To balance Vata, it is important to keep warm. Eat warm foods, especially foods that are sweet, sour, or salty. Drink Vata tea.

Vata colds generally include a dry cough, hoarseness, or laryngitis. A few drops of warmed sesame oil can be rubbed in the nasal passage to help soothe it. A Vata diet should be followed.

Pitta colds include a high fever and sore throat. A cooling Pitta routine should be followed.

Kapha colds and flus are those with a lot of mucus, runny nose, congestion, headache, and mild fever. Follow the Kapha routine and drink warm Kapha tea to help bring the body back into balance.

The following are some special Ayurvedic remedies for colds, cough, and sore throat:

→ **Throat Ease** Take 2 to 4 tablets at a time as often as needed.

→ **Cough Soothe: for Congestive Cough** Adults take 2 teaspoons twice a day; children should take 1 teaspoon twice daily.

→ **Cough Soothe: for Dry Cough** Adults take 2 teaspoons twice a day; children should take 1 teaspoon twice daily.

→ **Ayurvedic Balm** For temporary relief of minor aches and pains, apply a thin layer to affected area as often as needed.

→ BACH FLOWERS ←

Bach Flower remedies are a very safe and effective tool for treating colds and flu. The Bach Flowers system looks at the underlying cause of the cold symptoms. Often when our mind feels worn out, for whatever reason, our body also feels worn out, our immune system is weakened, and we are more likely to come down with a cold or the flu. Bach Flowers can help balance emotions and, therefore, prevent a cold or help you to relieve some of the causes of the cold, which, in turn, will help you get better. Lisa Marie's son Freddy is prone to ear infections when he gets a cold. She gives him Crab Apple several times a day to prevent them.

Here are some of the Bach Flower remedies that are helpful for the symptoms of colds and flu:

→ **Crab Apple** is a cleanser for mind and body.

→ **Hornbeam** helps strengthen a weary mind and body.

→ **Mustard** helps to fight depression.

→ **Olive** is useful when you feel fatigued or exhausted.

➤ **COLOR THERAPY** ◄

Specific color energies can target a variety of cold-related symptoms.

➤ **Blue** is the color of the throat chakra and of communication. Problems with the throat or voice, such as laryngitis or a cough and even sneezing, can be greatly helped with a treatment of blue color energy. Gargling with blue-infused water (water placed under a blue gel or in a blue glass and set in the sun or under a light for 30 seconds) is especially effective for sore throats and laryngitis. You also can drink color-infused water; it is important for people who have a cold or the flu to drink a lot of water.

➤ **Magenta,** or bright pink, can settle your stomach if you are suffering from nausea or vomiting. It can also alleviate a headache. Pink lightbulbs in bedroom lamps can be very soothing.

➤ **Orange** is a warming color. It is good for treating the common cold. Orange-infused water is especially effective for achy symptoms due to a cold.

➤ **Red** treats a more severe cold.

➤ **Turquoise,** a blue-green combination, helps to bring down a fever. Placing a compress soaked in turquoise-infused water and keeping it fresh and cool will help.

➤ **HERBS** ◄

Because of the overuse of antibiotics these days, bacteria are becoming more and more antibiotic-resistant. This means that you have to take stronger and stronger doses to kill various bacteria. And if you continue to take antibiotics, they may not work for you when you really need them. Antibiotics attack bacteria, but we need certain bacteria in our bodies for digestion and elimination. When the antibiotics attack these bacteria, we can become sick in other ways. If you or your child must take antibiotics to fight a bacterial infection, protect the body's good bacteria by taking a supplement of "friendly" bacteria, acidophilus. Acidophilus is often added to milk or yogurt. It also comes in capsules that require refrigeration. If you or another family member is lactose intolerant, make sure you buy the dairy-free version.

Garlic has many medicinal properties and is great for fighting off colds. Add it to foods and soups, or bake it and eat it straight. It is a real treat on warm sourdough bread with a little olive oil!

Nature produces many natural medicines to help fight off a nasty cold or the flu:

→ **Chamomile** can ease an upset stomach. It is especially beneficial if taken as tea.

→ **Echinacea,** particularly when combined with goldenseal, is an excellent remedy to build up the immune system. It acts as a natural antibiotic and helps get rid of infection. Adults may prefer capsules, but echinacea also comes in drops, which are easier for children to take. A raspberry-flavored version may taste better to children.

→ **Horseradish root** helps to get rid of laryngitis.

→ **Licorice root** can help bronchitis, a cough, or sore throat. It has potent antiviral effects. Various teas have licorice root in them. The hot liquid also will help to loosen up congestion.

→ **Marshmallow** eases the pain of a sore throat.

→ **Slippery elm** helps lubricate a dry sore throat.
→ **White willow bark** is like a natural aspirin for a headache.

Most herbs come in capsules. Adults usually have no problem with them, but if they are too large for your child to swallow, break them open and mix the powder with some applesauce or jelly. Follow the instructions on the bottle for the number of capsules per day.

→ HOMEOPATHY ←

Homeopathy is so specific that if the remedy you choose is not working for you, you need to choose another remedy that will more closely address the problem. We offer some general recommendations for homeopathic remedies in this book, but you may need to look at your symptoms individually (for example, is it a dry cough or a persistent cough? What part of the head is the headache pain coming from?) and consult a homeopathic reference to find the right remedy. Dozens of books have been written about homeopathy. If you are interested in learning more about it, any of the homeopathy books listed in the bibliography would be a good place to start. Meanwhile, check the following list to find some of your options for treating a cold or flu. The dosages will vary depending on the strength of the medication, so be sure to check the bottle for directions.

Aconitum napellus: Used for headache.
Allium cepa: Used for colds, cough, headache, laryngitis, sore throat.
Antimonium tartaricum: Used for cough.
Arsenicum album: Used for colds, sore throat.

Belladonna: Used for fever, headache, sore throat.

Bryonia alba: Used for colds, cough, fever, headache.

Calcarea phosphorica: Used for headache.

Carbo vegetabilis: Used for cough.

Chamomilla: Used for fever.

Ferrum phosphoricum: Used for fever, headache, sore throat, cough.

Gelsemium: Used for summer colds, headache, sore throat.

Hepar sulphuris calcareum: Used for cough, sore throat.

Ignatia amara: Used for headache.

Ipecac: Used for nausea, cough, vomiting.

Mercurius vivus: Used for sore throat, colds.

Nux vomica: Used for headache, nausea, colds, cough.

Phosphorus: Used for laryngitis, colds, cough, nausea, vomiting.

Pulsatilla: Used for runny nose, colds, cough.

Rhus toxicodendron: Used for cough.

Ruta graveolens: Used for headache.

Spongia tosta: Used for cough, colds, sore throat.

Sulfur: Used for colds, nausea.

Veratrum album: Used for headache, nausea, vomiting, cough.

✦ MEDITATION ✦

When you or your child has a cold or the flu, breathing may be difficult. Meditations incorporating breathing techniques will help to clear the nasal passages, unclog the sinuses, and provide more energy and stamina. The meditation technique called Vipassana, discussed in Chapter 2, is perfect to use at this time.

⇥ YOGA ⇤

Two Yoga postures that you and your family may wish to add to your regular Yoga routine are the Bridge or Shoulder Pose and the Lion. These will help to prevent colds and flu as well as stimulate the flow of blood in the head, neck, and chest area, to help your whole family recover from colds and the flu.

BRIDGE OR SHOULDER POSE

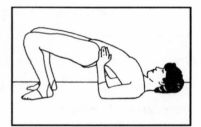

Basic Position:
Lie flat on your back with your knees bent and your feet about a shoulder-width apart. Keep your arms relaxed at your sides.

Instructions:
- ⇥ Slowly raise your buttocks and arch your back. Keep your heels on the floor, and place your hands firmly under your back for support. Your body should be supported by your feet, head, neck, shoulders, and upper arms.
- ⇥ Hold the posture as long as you comfortably can.
- ⇥ Slowly return to the basic position.
- ⇥ Repeat three to five times.
- ⇥ After your last stretch (to avoid back problems), lie on your back and hug your knees for a full minute more.

Breathing:
Inhale as you establish the position.
Breathe deeply while holding the posture.
Exhale as you return to your starting position.

Benefits:

Strengthens the arms, wrists, and lower back; limbers the spine; and builds resistance against colds.

THE LION

Basic position:

Sit cross-legged or in the half-lotus position (one foot on top of your thigh and the other tucked under your other thigh).

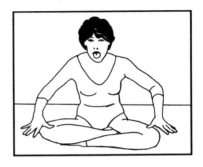

Instructions:

→ Place your hands over your knees with your fingers spread apart.

→ Extend your tongue outward and downward as far as you can.

→ At the same time, open your eyes wide.

→ Hold for as long as is comfortable.

→ Slowly return to the beginning position.

→ Repeat four times.

Breathing:

Inhale before starting the posture.

Exhale slowly while in the posture.

You also may produce a clear and steady

"*ah*" sound as you exhale.

Benefits:

Firms the muscles of the face and neck; sends extra blood to the throat; and massages and tones the neck muscles and ligaments.

5

Childhood Ailments
(That Make Kids Whiny)

K ids get all the same illnesses that adults do, but childhood comes with its own set of problems. First there's colic, then teething pain; each age brings something new.

In this chapter we suggest help for a variety of childhood ailments, including ear infections, chicken pox, asthma, bedwetting, measles, and hyperactivity. These home health remedies can help make your child more comfortable and your life easier.

We have listed the different types of remedies and therapies that can be easily administered for a variety of childhood ailments. In Appendix 1, we have compiled a list of therapies and remedies that can be used for specific symptoms. You may wish to look at the specific remedies for your child's symptoms first, but then be sure to check the discussion in the text for information about administering each of the remedies.

⤖ **ACUPRESSURE** ⤕

One reason why people, young and old, contract illness or just plain don't feel well is that their bodies' energy is out of balance or not evenly distributed. Blocks in the body can also inhibit the free flow of energy. Acupressure can help redistribute the body's energy and unblock blockages.

Use the acupressure points that follow for 1 to 2 minutes each, and repeat them each day until your energy or your child's energy seems more balanced. As always, the points are easy for children to use on themselves, but they must use firm and steady pressure. You can stimulate these points on yourself while encouraging your child. In this way, you bring yourself into balance as you help your child.

Be sure to stimulate the points on both sides of the body or directly on the midline of your body. Pressure can be applied while you are sitting or lying down.

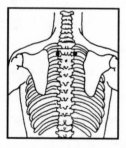

1ST UPPER BACK POINT
(Bladder 12)

Located just off of the second thoracic vertebra and next to the spine.

Benefits:
Useful for prevention of aches and pains and the remaining weakness of chills, fever, and flu.

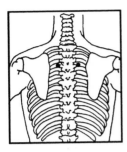

2ND UPPER BACK POINT
(Bladder 13)

Located on the edge of the spine, next to the third thoracic vertebra.

Benefits:
Useful for cough, congestion, agitation, boredom, and asthma.

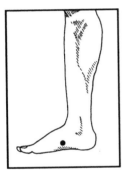

ARCH POINT
(Spleen 4)

Located in the arch of the inside foot, slightly behind the center of the arch. *Do not use on pregnant women.*

Benefits:
Useful for fever, body aches, upset stomach, cold feet, and diarrhea.

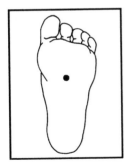

BOTTOM OF FOOT POINT
(Kidney 1)

Located in the depression one-third of the way from the toes to the heel, on the bottom of the foot. *Do not use on pregnant women.*

Benefits:
Useful for sore throat, head congestion, cold feet, weak energy.

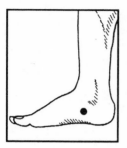

ANKLE POINT

(Kidney 2)

Located on the back upper edge of the arch on the inside of the foot. *Do not use on pregnant women.*

Benefits:

Useful for sore throat, head congestion, cold feet, weakness.

→ AROMATHERAPY ←

Any of the following oils can be used to help improve the symptoms of childhood ailments:

→ **Chamomile** can be used for sore throats or tonsillitis. It is also helpful for teething. Like lavender, it can relieve the itching of chicken pox and can be used instead of or in combination with lavender in the bath or lotion.

→ **Lavender** is used for earaches and ear infections. Add some to tea tree oil and massage the area just in front of the ear as well as just below the earlobe. Gently heat the mixture and apply to a cotton cloth to make a compress for the cheek and ear area. Lavender can also be used on a compress over the throat area to help sore throats and tonsillitis. For chicken pox, add lavender to calamine lotion to relieve itching. Or make a bath of lavender and baking soda and soak.

→ **Tea tree oil** is excellent for infections and can ease the pain of an earache. Apply 2 drops to a cotton ball and insert gently in the ear. Encourage whoever has the earache to breathe deeply.

→ **Thyme** can be added to the lavender/tea tree oil mixture for ear infections.

→ AYURVEDA ←

A fever generally comes from a Pitta imbalance. Any heat or redness from an infection can be cooled down with a Pitta routine. This includes a change in diet, exercise, and periods of quieting yourself or your child down through meditation. See Chapter 2 for meditation techniques.

Chapter 2 presents the complete routine for a Pitta imbalance. It also contains information necessary to understand the balance of all three mind/body types.

→ BACH FLOWERS ←

The following Bach Flower remedies are helpful for childhood ailments:

→ **Agrimony** can be used to alleviate asthma.

→ **Cherry Plum** is effective to help a child overcome bedwetting.

→ **Crab Apple** is a cleanser helpful with any kind of infection, including the ear infections so common in childhood.

→ **Holly** can be used to ease sibling rivalry.

→ **Walnut** is good for the advancing stages of life and could be used when children are teething or going through growing pains.

✦ COLOR THERAPY ✦

The following two colors are helpful in calming down symptoms of childhood problems:

✦ **Green** is a calming color most often used for healing. It can be used anytime you want to cool down an inflamed or infected area.
✦ **Blue** also can be used for helping earaches or the mumps.

✦ HERBS ✦

Many herbs are beneficial for childhood problems. The following are especially effective for many of the symptoms that come up at various stages of childhood:

✦ **Bearberry** is helpful in preventing bedwetting. You don't want to give the child too much liquid, so try to find the capsule form rather than bearberry tea. The capsule can be taken with a little water or swallowed with a spoonful of applesauce. Give the correct dosage indicated on the bottle right after dinner.
✦ **Chamomile** helps a child to sleep, calms an upset stomach, and makes a child with measles more comfortable. It can be taken in tea form, hot or iced with a little honey, or in capsules.
✦ **Melissa,** particularly when taken with passionflower, helps to calm a hyperactive child. It can be taken as a tea or in capsule form.
✦ **Mullein flower,** which often comes in oil drops, can be used to ease an earache. Place 2 drops on a cotton ball and insert gently in the ear.

→ **Passionflower** is calming and pain-relieving. Calming benefits are increased when it is taken as a warm tea.

→ HOMEOPATHY ←

The following homeopathic remedies are commonly used for various childhood ailments:

Aconitum napellus: Used for earache, colic.

Antimonium tartaricum: Used for chicken pox.

Belladonna: Used for earache, colic.

Calcarea phosphorica: Used for teething, growing pains.

Chamomilla: Used for earache, toothache, teething, colic.

Ferrum phosphoricum: Used for earache.

Magnesium phosphorica: Used for colic.

Mercurius vivus: Used for earache.

Pulsatilla: Used for earache, bedwetting, chicken pox.

Rhus toxicodendron: Used for chicken pox.

→ MEDITATION ←

When children don't feel well, they may not feel like meditating. Two meditations that may help to distract them from their symptoms are Tratak (Gazing) and the meditation of Listening, which includes listening to music, chanting, or natural sounds. Chapter 2 provides the details for these meditation techniques.

✣ YOGA ✣

The basic Yoga routine described in Chapter 2 should be done on a daily basis or a minimum of three times a week. It includes the Complete Breath, the Fish, and the Plow postures, all of which have very beneficial effects on childhood ailments. The following Pose of the Child posture is extremely beneficial for childhood ailments in particular. Help your child do this posture at least once a day when he or she is not feeling well.

POSE OF A CHILD

Basic Position:

✣ Kneel on the floor.

Instructions:

✣ Relax your whole body and close your eyes.

✣ Drop your forehead to the floor and relax all the muscles in your neck, back, and stomach.

✣ Relax your arms and legs.

✣ Remain in the posture for 2 or 3 minutes.

✣ Slowly return to the basic position.

✣ Repeat during your practice whenever you wish.

Breathing:

Exhale slowly while bending forward.

Breathe deeply while in the posture.

Inhale as you return to the basic position.

Benefits:

Massages the abdominal organs and separates the vertebrae slightly, which allows the spinal nerves to be stretched and toned gently. It is an excellent relaxation posture.

6

Cuts, Scrapes, Bumps, and Bruises

Many little mishaps can be treated at home with some TLC and a bandage. Here are some things you can do for the little problems to help yourself or family members heal more quickly and relieve body trauma. Remember, deep cuts may require stitches and a tetanus shot or booster. Consult a doctor immediately. Also, a physician should check any bump that looks unreasonably large.

⇥ ACUPRESSURE ⇤

Acupressure points are trigger spots for releasing muscle cramps. You can apply pressure directly on the muscle cramp itself, or you can press a series of specific points that are especially effective for muscle cramps or spasms. In either case, use steady, firm pressure or a counterclockwise massage. Pressure should be maintained or the massage continued for 2 or 3 minutes. If you have the stamina, your steady pressure will win out over the cramping muscle. When children get a cramp, their reflex is to tense up, which only makes the cramp worse. Your soothing voice will help to keep them calm and relax their muscles.

To keep the body in balance when using the following points, apply pressure to both sides of the body. Repeat the pressure every hour if the cramping persists.

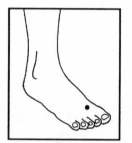

1ST TOP OF FOOT POINT
(Liver 3)

At the place where the first and second metatarsal bones meet. *Do not use on pregnant women.*

Benefits:
Useful for muscle cramps, spasms, cramping toes, weak feet, and fatigue.

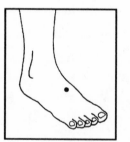

2ND TOP OF FOOT POINT
(Stomach 42)

On the top of the foot at the protrusion of the second metatarsal bone (above 2nd toe).

Benefits:
Useful for disorientation, chills, stomach upset.

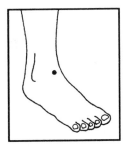

ANKLE CREASE POINT

(Stomach 41)

On the top of the foot at the ankle crease, above the second toe.

Benefits:

Useful for fear or agitation, numb muscles, cramping, stomach upset.

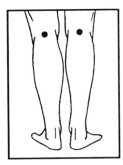

BEHIND THE KNEE POINT

(Bladder 54)

In the middle of the crease, at the back of the knee.

Benefits:

Useful for spasms, feeling cold, backache, pain in knee and back of leg.

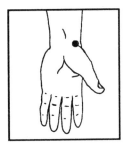

WRIST POINT

(Lung 9)

On the inside of the wrist, just above the thumb, in the major crease.

Benefits:

Useful for wrist pain, arm pain, shallow breathing.

✦ AROMATHERAPY ✦

Any of the following oils can be used for various skin conditions. Soak a soft cloth with cool water that has been infused with the oil and apply to the injury for about 15 minutes.

* **Chamomile** is excellent for bruises or bumps.
* **Geranium** is great for blisters and bruises.
* **Lavender** helps prevent bug bites and also can help the itchiness if you already have a bite. Lavender helps speed the healing of bruises, bumps, and burns. It also can help with cuts, especially when used in combination with tea tree oil in a warm-water bath.
* **Thyme** can be used in combination with lavender to prevent bug bites or promote the healing of bites you already have.

✦ AYURVEDA ✦

Pitta mind/body types are more prone to skin disorders, as Pitta governs complexion. Most skin problems can be treated with a Pitta routine of diet and exercise. A full explanation of this routine is given in Chapter 2.

Within the Ayurvedic system, ghee, or clarified butter, is used to treat skin problems. You will find ghee in the refrigerated section of a health food store. Ghee is an excellent external treatment for rashes, burns, and inflammatory skin diseases. It should be diluted with water to half strength and kept, preferably, in a copper container for a month to make it more absorbable for the skin.

A Pitta imbalance can cause a skin disease characterized by

redness, swelling, and infection. People with these problems should avoid exposure to the sun and heat and follow the Pitta routine.

A Vata imbalance can cause a skin disease that is dry, itchy, or scaly. If these are your symptoms, you should avoid the wind, use a soothing sesame oil massage and follow the Vata routine.

A Kapha imbalance can cause a skin disease with oozing or weeping sores. People with this problem should avoid oils, dampness, and cold and follow the Kapha routine.

→ BACH FLOWERS ←

Louise always keeps Rescue Remedy cream in her kitchen and in her handbag for all kinds of minor emergencies. Here are Bach Flower remedies that are helpful for skin problems:

→ **Crab Apple** can help clear up acne or heal a rash.
→ **Star of Bethlehem** is useful after a bug bite or bee sting when you feel woozy or go into a state of shock.
→ **Rescue Remedy** cream can be applied to the skin for all kinds of problems, including burns, cuts, and bug bites. This ointment helps wounds or bruises to heal much faster.

→ COLOR THERAPY ←

The following color therapy suggestions can be used for skin conditions:

→ **Blue** is useful for most skin conditions. It can cool down any burn, including a sunburn. It can help heal bruises, blisters, sores, and sprains.

→ **Green** helps to get rid of warts.

→ **Turquoise** helps improve acne and cold sores. It also eases the sting of insect bites.

→ **Violet** is also effective on warts.

→ HERBS ←

During the summer, Lisa Marie keeps extra aloe vera gel on hand for sunburn pain. It's nongreasy and doesn't smell, so her kids don't complain when she puts it on their burns.

The following herbs can be used for various skin conditions:

→ **Aloe vera** comes in a gel and is also often added to ointments. A natural moisturizer, it is a traditional remedy that speeds the healing of the skin, including cuts and some types of acne.

→ **Calendula** comes in a cream or oil and helps to heal bruises.

→ **Goldenseal** mixed with water can be applied directly to the skin to help clear up acne.

→ **St. John's Wort oil,** applied topically, heals burns, bruises, and other wounds.

→ **Thuja leaf oil,** applied topically, helps get rid of warts.

⇒ HOMEOPATHY ⇐

The following homeopathic remedies can help with various skin problems:

Antimonium tartaricum: Used for acne.

Apis mellifica: Used for bee stings, insect bites, swelling.

Arnica montana: Used for bruises, sore muscles. (Arnica also comes in a gel or cream form that can be applied topically.)

Cantharis: Used for burns, sunburn, stings.

Hepar sulphuris calcareum: Used for insect bites.

Hypericum: Used for puncture wounds, bites, bee stings, burns.

Ledum palustre: Used for bites, stings, puncture wounds, sprains, bruises.

Rhus toxicodendron: Used for sprains, strains, sore muscles, cold sores, poison ivy, hives.

Ruta graveolens: Used for sprains.

Sulfur: Used for acne.

⇒ MEDITATION ⇐

After the body tenses up from injury, meditation is a very powerful and natural way to help you or your child calm down and return to a state of ease. Any meditation technique that includes deep breathing will help to calm the mind and release bodily tension. See Chapter 2 for meditation styles that are most appropriate for you or your child.

⟶ YOGA ⟵

Yoga is used for reestablishing the balance of energy after the pain or discomfort of being injured. If you do some Yoga shortly after an injury, the body will return to its normal state very quickly. After trauma has set into the muscles and the body has absorbed the memory of the injury, rebalancing takes considerably more effort.

The following three Yoga postures will help rebalance the body after injury:

POSE OF A CHILD
(described on page 96)

THE COMPLETE BREATH
(described on page 43)

UPRIGHT HEAD-TO-KNEE POSE
(described on page 72)

7

Sleeplessness

The night seems endlessly long when you can't get to sleep. And the day after a sleepless night is never fun. Sleep is important to your health in many ways. It allows your body and mind to rest and replenish for times of activity. Following are some remedies that can help get you or your child over sleeplessness.

✦ ACUPRESSURE ✦

Inability to get to sleep or to stay asleep can be caused by emotional and mental tension. It is often said that insomnia is caused by uneven distribution of energy, when there is excess energy in some areas of the body and not enough in others. The acupressure points on the sides of the heels are very effective for sleeplessness. The points on the head help to calm your thoughts and emotions and allow you to go to sleep.

If possible, press these points daily on yourself or your child, at least 30 minutes before bedtime. Press them on both sides of the body. The point on the top of the head should be pressed in the very midline on top of the head.

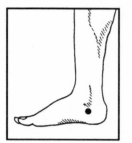

INNER ANKLE POINT
(Kidney 6)

In the depression located one thumb's width below the inner ankle bone. *Do not use on pregnant women.*

Benefits:
Useful for insomnia, restlessness, stage fright, fear of the dark.

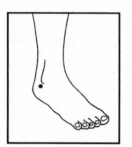

OUTER ANKLE POINT
(Bladder 62)

In the depression underneath the outer ankle bone.

Benefits:
Useful for insomnia, tension headache; promotes relaxed sleep.

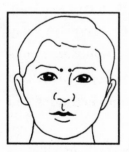

EYEBROW POINT
(Bladder 2)

In the depression at the inner corner of the eyebrow.

Benefits:
Useful for insomnia, brain-tiredness, headache, eye tension.

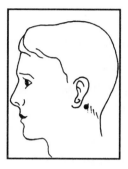

NECK POINT

(Special Point)

One inch behind the bottom of the earlobe.

Benefits:

Useful for insomnia, neck ache, headache, nausea.

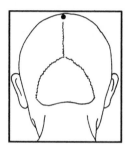

TOP OF HEAD POINT

(Governing Vessel 20)

At the point where a line drawn up from the top of the ear crosses the center line of the top of the head.

Benefits:

Useful for headache, insomnia.

↛ AROMATHERAPY ↚

Any of the following oils can help you get to sleep. Louise keeps an aroma pot filled with lavender on her nightstand to help her sleep peacefully. If you place 6 to 8 drops of one of the following aromas in a warm bath, you'll be prepared for a restful night's sleep. You also can place 3 to 4 drops of one of the essential oils on a light ring or in an aroma diffuser in your bedroom or your child's.

- ↛ **Chamomile**
- ↛ **Lavender**
- ↛ **Sandalwood**

⇢ AYURVEDA ⇠

Vata mind/body types often have difficulty falling asleep or staying asleep. Their minds are active, imaginative, and restless and may be hard to quiet down at night. Kapha mind/body types need a lot of sleep, or they become groggy and ineffective.

Ayurveda recommends that everyone keep a regular bedtime and morning routine. Bedtime should be at the same time each night, preferably by 10:00 P.M. for adults. Children need more sleep and should be in bed earlier. The hours before bed should be spent in quiet activity, Yoga, and meditation. Adults and children should awaken at dawn, between 6:00 A.M. and 8:00 A.M., and proceed with their daily rituals.

Vata tea (containing the herbs licorice, ginger, cardamom, and cinnamon) is calming and aids in a good night's sleep. A warm sesame oil massage followed by a warm bath or shower is also very relaxing and will help you get to sleep.

⇢ BACH FLOWERS ⇠

Bach Flowers can be a very safe and effective tool in treating insomnia. When using Bach Flower remedies for sleeping problems, you should look at the cause of your trouble to find the proper remedy.

⇢ **Agrimony** is useful for general insomnia, when you're not sure what's causing it.

→ **Oak** is effective when you are struggling against your tiredness.

→ **Olive** is used when you are completely exhausted.

→ **White Chestnut** helps get rid of those recurring thoughts that keep you awake at night.

→ COLOR THERAPY ←

Cool colors—blue, green, turquoise, and violet—are calming. If you or your children are having trouble sleeping, your environment may be too stimulating. Use cool colors in your decor, in your sheets, and in your nightclothes. Surround yourself with plants and peace, and your body will be more relaxed, enabling you to drift off to sleep.

→ HERBS ←

The following herbs are helpful for insomnia and for more restful sleep:

→ **Chamomile,** particularly as a hot tea, is a traditional sleep remedy.

→ **Passionflower** is calming. It is readily available in capsule form. If your child cannot swallow the capsule, break it open and mix the powder with a little applesauce or jelly.

→ **Valerian** is a strong sleep-inducer. It is best for adults or older children. While it does come in a tea, because of its strong flavor you and your children may prefer to take it in capsule form.

⇥ HOMEOPATHY ⇤

Lisa Marie uses a combination of belladonna and chamomilla when her son Freddy is restless and cannot sleep. The following homeopathic remedies are recommended for insomnia or sleeplessness:

⇥ *Belladonna* is helpful when you're sleepy but can't sleep.

⇥ *Chamomilla* is generally calming.

⇥ *Ferrum phosphoricum* is helpful when a headache is keeping you awake.

⇥ *Ignatia amara* is helpful when depression is keeping you awake.

⇥ *Nux vomica* is helpful when you wake up after 3:00 A.M. and can't get back to sleep.

⇥ *Pulsatilla* is helpful when it is difficult to get to sleep and then sleep is restless.

⇥ *Sulfur* helps you sleep when you keep waking up, especially between 2:00 A.M. and 5:00 A.M.

⇥ *Calms Forte* is a unique combination of several different homeopathic medicines that work gently to help you get to sleep and stay asleep.

⇥ MEDITATION ⇤

Meditation is an especially valuable tool for sleeplessness and also for getting restful sleep from which you wake up feeling refreshed and energetic. Meditation calms the mind, the body, and the emotions and balances the body's energy. Mantra Meditation and meditations using breath are extremely beneficial and easy for adults and children. Meditation should be practiced within one-half hour of bedtime. Afterward, there should be no further stimulation, such as watching TV or playing video games, before going to bed. See Chapter 2 for meditation techniques to help with sleep.

→ YOGA ←

One of the major benefits of doing Yoga on a regular basis is that it helps you relax and release the tensions of your body. When doing the following three postures, allow your body to relax and breathe deeply. These postures are especially beneficial for insomnia because they stimulate the acupressure points around the ankles and around the head, areas traditionally used to promote calm and deep sleep.

Practicing these postures daily until regular sleep patterns can be established will prove useful for adults and children.

POSE OF A CHILD
(described on page 96)

BRIDGE OR SHOULDER POSE
(described on page 86)

THE CAMEL

Basic position:
Kneel on the floor, knees and feet shoulder-width apart, arms at your sides.

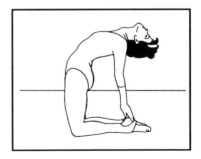

Instructions:

→ Carefully arch your back, and place your right hand on your right heel and your left hand on your left heel.

→ Arch your head back and press your hips forward.

→ Contract your buttock muscles and keep the weight of your body over your knees.

→ Remain in the stretch as long as you comfortably can.

→ Slowly return to the basic position.

→ Repeat up to five times.

→ After your last stretch (to avoid back problems), lie on your back and hug your knees to your chest for a full minute.

Breathing:

Inhale while in the basic position.

Exhale while bending backward.

Breathe normally while in the stretch.

Exhale while returning to the basic position.

Benefits:

Improves digestion and elimination, and strengthens the lower back, arms, and legs.

8

Stressed Out?

When you are feeling under stress, your body is not able to work at its maximum efficiency to keep you healthy. That is why stress is at the root of so many different, more serious diseases.

With our hectic lifestyles and busy schedules, it's hard not to be under stress these days! Even children, with school, homework, after-school activities, and peer pressure, feel stressed out at times.

To help relieve the stress in your family's life and enable you to be more at peace, we've found these remedies to be useful.

⤑ ACUPRESSURE ⤐

Acupressure is especially beneficial for feelings of stress and inability to cope, because it is such a powerful way to relax and rebalance your body. The following points will help you remain centered. Louise uses them on most of her clients at the Healing Arts Center because so many people are leading stressful lives today.

Each point can be done individually, or they can all be done as a group. Do them on a daily basis and hold each point for about 2 minutes. Help your children do the points at first.

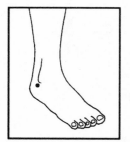

OUTER ANKLE POINT

(Bladder 62)

In the depression underneath the outer ankle bone.

Benefits:

Useful for nervousness, tension headaches.

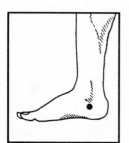

INNER ANKLE POINT

(Kidney 6)

In the depression located one thumb's width below the inner ankle bone. *Do not use on pregnant women.*

Benefits:

Useful for insomnia, headaches.

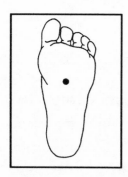

BOTTOM OF FOOT POINT

(Kidney 1)

Located in the depression one-third of the way from the toes to the heel, on the bottom of the foot.

Do not use on pregnant women.

Benefits:

Useful for centering and energy balance.

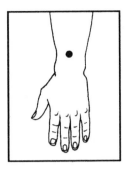

BACK OF WRIST POINT

(Triple Warmer 5)

About 2 inches up from the back of the wrist, between the two bones of the forearm.

Benefits:

Useful for relieving hypertension, depression, headache, or nervousness.

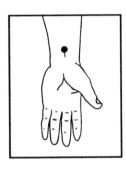

2ND WRIST POINT

(Pericardium 6)

On the inside of the arm, about 2 inches up from the crease of the wrist, between the two large bones of the forearm.

Do not use on pregnant women.

Benefits:

Useful for relieving depression, dizziness, nausea, nervousness, sleepiness.

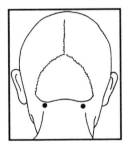

BASE OF SKULL POINT

(Gallbladder 20)

Just below the occipital bone and 2 inches from the midline of the neck.

Benefits:

Useful for relieving fear and aggression.

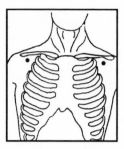

FRONT SHOULDER POINT
(Lung 1)

On the front of the chest wall, 1 inch below the clavicle and 6 inches out from the sternum.

Benefits:
Useful for letting go of frustration, fear, or anger.

→ AROMATHERAPY ←

Any of these oils can be used to help you calm down and feel more relaxed:

→ **Basil** is good in the workplace, as it helps with environmental and mental stress.

→ **Chamomile** is calming when you feel stressed from the environment, loud noises, or uncomfortable arrangements. It also is used when you feel physically stressed, as from a long commute or from working out too much.

→ **Geranium** is excellent for combating all kinds of stresses.

→ **Lavender** is good for physical or mental stress, or for chemical stress, as when you've drunk too much coffee or eaten too much junk food.

→ **Rose** is especially good for emotional stress.

→ AYURVEDA ←

Ojas is an Ayurvedic word that refers to our life energy. Translated, it means "vigor." Stress greatly reduces ojas, which then weakens the immune system. When ojas is low, disease can follow.

To replenish ojas, follow the routine for your mind/body type (see Chapter 3). Some foods, such as milk and ghee, are especially good for increasing ojas. Meditation is the best thing you can do to alleviate stress and thereby increase ojas.

Vata tea is calming and soothes the nerves. It is delicious with a little bit of brown sugar.

If you're feeling stressed because you are angry, Pitta tea will help "cool you off."

→ BACH FLOWERS ←

Bach Flowers are extremely powerful in fighting and even preventing stress. Most stress has an emotional basis, and Bach Flowers are excellent for getting to that emotion.

→ **Aspen** should be taken when you feel a vague foreboding, when your fear is from an unknown origin.

→ **Impatiens** helps to relieve mental and physical tension. It should be used when you feel irritable or impatient.

→ **Mimulus** soothes nerves. It is best used when you have a fear of something known.

→ **Red Chestnut** is helpful when you fear for someone else's health or safety.

→ **Rock Rose** alleviates extreme fear and panic attacks.

→ **Rock Water** helps you to relax when you overwork or are hard on yourself.

→ **Vervain** helps to relieve the stress and tension you feel from overenthusiasm and overeffort.

→ **White Chestnut** is best for getting rid of worry and unwanted thoughts.

→ COLOR THERAPY ←

Specific energies respond significantly to a variety of stress symptoms. Stress goes with you wherever you go, and your environment has a strong influence on how stressed you feel. The color of your clothes and the colors in your home and workplace have a strong effect on your mood and tension level. Wear and surround yourself with colors that make you feel more at peace. Placing cool-colored lightbulbs in your lamp will also bring down your stress level.

→ **Blue** is calming and helps to relieve anxiety.

→ **Orange** is a mood lifter and will help you to overcome fatigue or depression.

→ **Turquoise** alleviates stress and tension.

HERBS ←

The following herbs can help reduce the stress level in your life:

→ **Melissa** is calming and is best used in combination with passionflower.

→ **Passionflower** is calming and helps to relieve anxiety.

→ **Skullcap** reduces stress and relieves anxiety.

→ **Valerian** reduces stress but also can make you sleepy.

→ HOMEOPATHY ←

The following homeopathic remedies can be used effectively to alleviate stress:

Arsenicum album: Used for anxiety.

Gelsemium: Used for stage fright.

Ignatia amara: Used for emotional strain, mental stress.

Phosphorus: Used for anxiety.

Calms Forte: A combination of homeopathic medicines used for nervous tension and for insomnia.

→ MEDITATION ←

Meditation is the single most important way that you can reduce stress in your life. A regular 20-minute meditation routine in the morning and before bed will clear your mind and deeply relax your body. This, in turn, helps to lower your heart rate, relax your muscles, improve your breathing, and bring your stress level down. It will also help you gain valuable insights and allow you to understand yourself better. If a 20-minute meditation does not fit into your schedule, 5-minute meditations throughout the day will also give you great benefits. Use any of the meditation styles described in Chapter 2. Note that it is valuable to change your meditation style each day to keep your meditation practice fresh and interesting. Frequent changes in style will also help to keep your child interested. You may wish to encourage your child to meditate by practicing with him or her until it becomes a habit. Children often enjoy soft music in the background when they meditate.

✦ YOGA ✦

Yoga is a powerful way of toning the nervous system. Through the movement, stretching, breathing, and relaxation, Yoga provides a deep release of tension and relaxes the entire body. The following Yoga postures can be done together as a routine that will allow the spine to stretch and then relax. Ending the routine with the Complete Breath pose will release in the body a sense of calm and revitalization. While these postures are fun for children to do, you may wish to practice them along with your children or help them to do the postures correctly until they perfect them.

THE COMPLETE BREATH
(described on page 43)

BRIDGE OR SHOULDER POSE
(described on page 86)

SPINAL ROCK

Basic position:

Sit on the floor.

Clasp your arms around your knees, or sit cross-legged and hold onto your feet.

Instructions:

→ Be sure your knees remain bent throughout the exercise.

→ Holding your initial position, roll backward on your back as far as you comfortably can.

→ Keep your chin tucked toward your chest and your back slightly rounded.

→ Maintaining your momentum, roll forward to a seated position.

→ Repeat five to seven times, maintaining a gentle rocking motion.

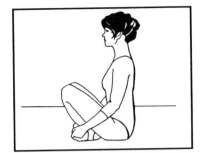

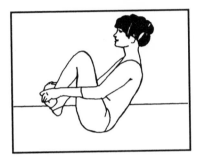

Breathing:

Inhale in the basic position.
Exhale while rocking backward.
Inhale while rocking forward.

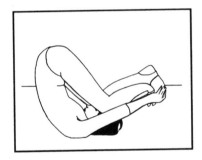

Limitations:

Do not do this asana if you have spinal problems or are menstruating heavily.

Benefits:

Warms up your muscles, limbers the spine, and inverts blood flow; excellent toning for the entire body.

CORPSE POSE

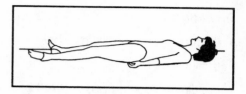

Basic position:

Lie flat on your back with your
arms beside your body, palms
facing upward. Move your feet slightly apart to a comfortable position and
close your eyes.

Instructions:

→ Relax your whole body.

Breathing:

Concentrate on your breath and let it become rhythmic and natural.
Become aware of the inhalation and exhalation.
If your mind starts to wander, bring it back to the breath.
By focusing your mind on your breath for just a few minutes, a state
of deep relaxation will occur.

Benefits:

Relaxes your entire body, especially when combined with deep breathing.

9

Digestion (and Plumbing Problems)

Many digestive problems, such as upset stomach, come from stress. If stress is the root of your digestive problems, reread Chapter 8 for ways to relax.

Irritable bowel syndrome is a common digestive problem characterized by alternating constipation and diarrhea. This is more common in adults but can occur in children as well. One typical symptom is the stomach feeling crampy a few hours after eating. Mild symptoms of irritable bowel syndrome can be controlled by choosing appropriate foods and by using some of the natural remedies discussed here. If, however, the symptoms persist or worsen, you need to see a physician.

Irritable bowel syndrome has been likened to diabetes of the colon. The colon is particularly sensitive to various sugars. If you suspect that you or your child has this syndrome, try eliminating lactose, or milk sugar, from the diet. Lactose is found in milk, cream, and ice cream but is not in cheese, yogurt, or butter. The enzyme in the colon that breaks down lactose is usually the first to be affected by stress.

Many people are lactose intolerant. Lactose-free milk and cream are readily available at most markets now.

If a lactose-free diet doesn't solve the problem, try eliminating citrus and then corn products, including anything containing corn syrup. Lettuce and other high-fiber fresh vegetables, fruits, and nuts, as well as beef products, are also hard to digest and can bring on symptoms. If eliminating these foods doesn't work, you may have *celiac sprue,* which is an intolerance to wheat. See your doctor for a thorough checkup.

Sorbitol and manitol, which are often found in gum, candy, and breath fresheners, are also colon irritants and should be avoided. It is important to read the labels on the foods you buy and know what you are eating. By doing so, you'll be able to find out what is eating you!

Commercial laxatives are a temporary solution for constipation, but not a very good one. Some chemicals in laxatives can aggressively deplete the colon of the natural bacteria that it needs for elimination. So laxatives end up aggravating your condition. When constipated, try foods that have a natural laxative effect: prunes and prune juice, and products containing a high amount of bran. You should also drink a minimum of 64 ounces of water a day. This in itself can often act as a natural laxative.

A natural diet to help relieve diarrhea is called the BRAT diet, which is especially effective for children. BRAT stands for "bananas, rice, applesauce, and toast." These foods all have properties to control diarrhea.

Besides diet, here are some other ways that you can improve digestive problems.

→ ACUPRESSURE ←

Acupressure stimulates the flow of energy, which can improve digestion and help with problems such as constipation and diarrhea. Use these acupressure points when problems occur; if you use them daily, they can regulate the body so that the digestive problems are kept to a minimum.

Press them on both sides of the body for about 2 minutes each. Assist your child in maintaining steady pressure. After learning the points, your child can do them by him- or herself.

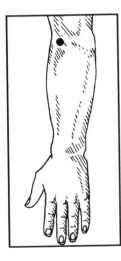

ELBOW POINT
(Large Intestine 11)

At the outside end of the elbow crease when the elbow is bent at 90 degrees. Press against the bone.

Benefits:
Useful for constipation, gas pains.

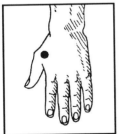

BACK OF HAND POINT
(Large Intestine 4)

On the back of the hand, between the thumb and first finger. *Do not use on pregnant women.*

Benefits:
Useful for diarrhea, constipation, headaches, gas.

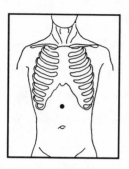

ABDOMEN POINT

(Conception Vessel 12)

Halfway between the navel and the bottom of the sternum, on the midline of the abdomen.

Benefits:

Useful for stomach upset, gas, stomach pain.

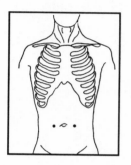

OUT FROM NAVEL POINT

(Stomach 25)

About 1 inch out from the navel.

Benefits:

Useful for gas, constipation.

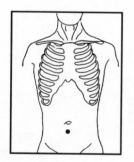

LOWER ABDOMEN POINT

(Conception Vessel 6)

About 2 inches below the navel, on the midline of the body.

Benefits:

Useful for upset stomach, digestion, gas; increases energy.

→ AROMATHERAPY ←

Any of these oils can be used to help improve discomfort associated with digestion:

→ **Chamomile** helps ease diarrhea. You can wear the oil as a perfume. You can also make a massage oil by diluting 6 drops of the essential oil in 1/4 cup of neutral carrier oil, such as sesame or safflower oil. Massage onto the lower abdomen after each bout with diarrhea.

→ **Ginger** is excellent for digestive problems. It can be used as a massage oil by diluting 6 drops in 1/4 cup of carrier oil. Massage the stomach clockwise to help regulate the intestine, whether the problem is constipation or diarrhea.

→ **Patchouli** can be used in the same way as ginger, as a massage oil, to clean the intestines. It is commonly found in incense.

→ **Peppermint** helps when you have indigestion or a nervous stomach. It also alleviates gas. Wear it as a perfume or carry around a cotton ball with a few drops on it in your pocket.

→ **Sandalwood** is used to treat diarrhea. It can be used in a massage oil. Some aromatic soaps are made with sandalwood.

→ AYURVEDA ←

Ayurveda teaches that good digestion leads to good health and that poor digestion can bring disease. Each mind/body type digests differently. When planning your meals, it is important to understand your mind/body type and how it digests food.

Vata digestion varies and can be delicate. Vatas should favor warm foods with moderately heavy textures. Foods should include salty, sour, and sweet tastes.

Pitta digestion is usually strong and intense. Pittas should favor cool or warm, rather than hot, foods with moderately heavy textures. Foods should include bitter, sweet, and astringent tastes.

Kapha digestion is slower and heavier. Kaphas should favor warm, light food. Food should be as dry as possible, cooked without much water. Tastes should be pungent, bitter, and astringent. Kaphas prefer spicy food, which promotes better digestion for them.

Agni is an Ayurvedic term meaning "digestive fire." When agni is in good supply, you feel good, your digestion is strong. To increase agni, it is best to eat meals at the same time each day. Breakfast should be light, lunch fairly substantial, and dinner light and eaten early.

→ **Ghee,** or clarified butter, is great for increasing agni and restoring proper digestion.

→ **Ginger,** as a tea or as a spice, is commonly used for poor digestion or to increase appetite.

→ **Cloves, cinnamon,** and **black pepper** are recommended to aid in digestion.

Ayurveda offers the following guidelines to everyone who wants to improve his or her digestion:

→ Sit down while you eat. Eat in a quiet atmosphere. Focus on the food; do not read or watch TV as you eat.

→ Don't rush through meals or linger over them too long.

→ Eat meals at approximately the same times every day.

→ Stop eating before you are completely full.

→ Allow approximately 3 to 6 hours between meals for digestion.

→ Eat when you are hungry, when the stomach is empty.

→ Sip warm water or juice with meals. Drink milk separately from meals, either alone or with other sweet foods.

→ Avoid ice-cold food and beverages.

→ Sit quietly for a few minutes after eating.

→ BACH FLOWERS ←

When you or a family member is having digestive problems, you need to look at the cause behind those problems. Many digestive problems are stress-related. If this is the case for you, see Chapter 8 for some additional suggestions.

→ **Crab Apple** is a cleanser and can be used to help clear up constipation.

→ **Holly** is used when you are angry.

→ **Mimulus** is for when you know you are afraid of something.

→ **Walnut** is used when you are making changes in your life.

→ **Wild Chestnut** is used when you continually worry.

⇥ COLOR THERAPY ⇤

Use color therapy to infuse specific energies for various digestive problems.

⇥ **Blue** helps to calm a nervous stomach. Twice daily, drink 4 ounces of water that has been infused with the blue vibration.

⇥ **Magenta** helps to relieve nausea or vomiting. Drape a magenta scarf over a lampshade and take deep breaths, envisioning the magenta color being infused into your body.

⇥ **Orange** is a stimulating color used to alleviate constipation. Twice daily, drink 4 ounces of water that has been infused with the orange vibration.

⇥ HERBS ⇤

The following herbs are helpful with digestive problems:

⇥ **Aloe vera** is a stimulant laxative. This herb is available only in capsule form. The capsule may be opened and its contents mixed in applesauce or jelly if swallowing it is a problem.

⇥ **Cascara sagrada** acts as a laxative. This herb is available in capsule form and is better for adults and older children.

Lisa Marie's son Brian enjoys a sweet chamomile tea when he has an upset stomach. The following herbs are found in tea or capsule form and can be taken either way:

→ **Chamomile** relieves a digestive headache.

→ **Ginger** aids digestion and calms diarrhea.

→ **Peppermint** helps ease indigestion.

→ **Red raspberry,** which comes either as leaves or as root bark, helps get rid of diarrhea.

→ HOMEOPATHY ←

The following homeopathic remedies help to correct digestive problems:

Arsenicum album: Used for diarrhea.

Bryonia alba: Used for constipation, diarrhea.

Cantharis: Used for indigestion.

Chamomilla: Used for diarrhea.

China: Used for gas.

Ipecac: Used for diarrhea.

Mercurius vivus: Used for diarrhea.

Nux vomica: Used for indigestion, constipation with diarrhea.

Phosphorus: Used for diarrhea, constipation.

Pulsatilla: Used for indigestion.

Sulfur: Used for diarrhea, constipation.

Veratrum album: Used for constipation, diarrhea.

→ MEDITATION ←

Poor digestion is often a signal that the body is in need of relaxation, centering, and balance. Meditation helps to bring the body into a state of centeredness and calmness. This in turn will help the body to digest food more thoroughly and to derive more nutrition from the foods eaten. Any of the meditation methods covered in Chapter 2 are useful. Try the breathing techniques especially and focus the breath in the abdominal cavity. Do the Complete Breath, as shown on page 43, and visualize the entire abdominal cavity, relaxing as you exhale. This technique is easy for children; they'll derive further benefit from their meditation if their parents practice the technique with them.

→ YOGA ←

By your stretching the body and the organs of digestion, new energy is released to improve digestion and all of the problems that occur in the gastrointestinal tract. Through the postures, energy can be released that aids in bringing the system to a healthier state. The postures can be done as needed or on a regular basis 2 to 3 times a week. Parents should watch their children to be sure the postures are being done correctly. For a healthier body, parents may also wish to join in.

THE CAMEL
(described on page 113)

THE WHEEL

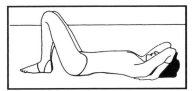

Basic position:

Lie on your back with your knees bent and your heels close to your buttocks. Rest your arms comfortably at your sides.

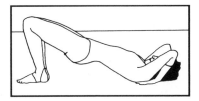

Instructions:

→ Bend your arms with elbows pointing toward the ceiling.

→ Place your fingertips underneath your shoulders.

→ Slowly raise your body in a straight line from your knees to your shoulders.

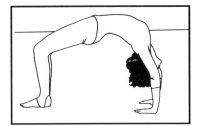

→ Using the strength of your arms, raise your shoulders off the floor and let the crown of your head rest on the floor to support the weight of your upper body.

→ Straighten your arms and legs, lift your head off the floor, and raise your body to a fully arched height.

→ Remain in the position as long as you comfortably can.

→ Slowly lower your body back to the head-based, then the supine, position.

→ Rather than repeating the Wheel several times, do it only once and hold it for as long as you can comfortably.

→ After your stretch (to avoid back problems), lie on your back and hug your knees for a full minute.

Benefits:

Strengthens back and arm muscles; tones arms, legs, waist, and spine; reverses blood flow; and aids in digestion and elimination.

THE LOCUST POSE

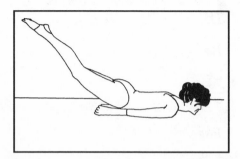

Basic position:

Lie on your stomach with your hands in a fist under your thighs to give leverage. Your chin should be touching the floor.

Instructions:

- ➔ Stretch your legs and tense your arms.
- ➔ Raise your legs as high as possible without bending them.
- ➔ Hold the position for as long as you wish.
- ➔ Slowly return to your original position.
- ➔ Repeat three to five times.

Breathing:

Inhale before you start.

Hold your breath while raising your legs.

Exhale while returning to the starting position.

Limitations:

Do not practice the Locust if you have an ulcer, hernia, or lower back problems.

Benefits:

Beneficial for all the abdominal organs, acts on the intestines aiding digestion and elimination, and strengthens the lower back.

THE BOW

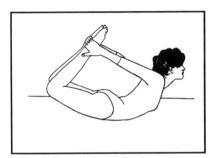

Basic position:

Lie flat on your stomach with your
arms at your sides.

Instructions:

→ Bend your knees and hold onto
  your ankles.

→ Arch your back.

→ Using the strength of your arm muscles, pull back on your ankles as
  you raise your head, chest, and thighs.

→ Look up as high as you can.

→ Be sure to keep your arms straight.

→ Hold the position as long as you comfortably can.

→ Slowly and carefully return to the basic position.

→ Repeat between three and five times.

→ After your last stretch, to avoid back problems, lie on your back and
  hug your knees for a full minute or more.

Breathing:

Inhale as you stretch into the posture.

Breathe deeply during the stretch.

Exhale as you slowly return to the basic position.

Limitations:

Do not practice the Bow if you have ulcers, hernia, or lower back pain.

Benefits:

Massages the abdominal organs and muscles, and aids digestion and elimination.

10

Concentration

Our mental health is essential to our overall physical health. When the mind is clear, alert, and focused, we process information more efficiently. We can learn more quickly and easily and improve our memory. This, in turn, increases confidence and promotes a positive attitude. And, of course, a healthy, positive attitude encourages a healthy lifestyle and a healthy body!

We are required to focus and concentrate at many times in our lives. One of these times is when we are in school. We've all experienced that falling-asleep-in-class phenomenon. A boring lecture acts as a sedative that lulls us into a state of unconsciousness, but we pay the price during final exams!

Children face this challenge every day in the classroom. No matter how intriguing the teacher's lesson may be, a child's active imagination often wins the battle for his or her attention.

In the business world, we need to keep our minds on our jobs in order to perform well. We've got to block out distractions, either internal or external, and focus on the task at hand.

At home, we've got to juggle several situations at a time and give each the attention it deserves. We make lists, keep appointment books, organize, schedule, and delegate. We have to keep track of who is going where with whom and when. There are phone calls to make, groceries to buy, dry cleaning to pick up, laundry to do, meals to make, homework to turn in, and pets to feed. Good mental function allows us to handle our busy lives with a minimum of stress.

Everyone has trouble focusing now and then, but when lack of concentration is an ongoing problem, you may suspect an attention disorder. Attention deficit disorder, or ADD, is a neurobiological disorder that affects approximately 3 to 5 percent of the school-age population. ADD is not a condition that is "outgrown." About two-thirds of those children identified with ADD continue to show symptoms into adulthood.

In studies performed at the National Institute of Mental Health, advanced brain-imaging techniques have shown that the frontal lobe of an ADD brain is chemically different from that of a non-ADD brain. The frontal lobe is important for attention, handwriting, motor control, and inhibition of responses.

ADD is a medical condition that is usually genetic. Typically, people with ADD are easily distracted, impulsive, and restless. The symptoms of ADD appear in early childhood, are ongoing, and are not caused by physical, emotional, or mental stress. If left undiagnosed or untreated, a child with ADD is at risk of having poor self-esteem, an impaired learning ability, social problems, and family conflicts.

Here are some other characteristics that a person with ADD may exhibit:

→ fidgeting with hands or feet

→ difficulty remaining seated

→ difficulty following through on instructions

→ shifting from one uncompleted task to another

→ difficulty playing or working quietly

→ interrupting

→ daydreaming at inappropriate times

→ participating in dangerous activities

→ mood swings

→ disorganized work space, living area

→ impatience

→ insatiability, a feeling of never being satisfied

People with ADD usually are bright, creative, and have a sparkling sense of humor. But because of their behavior, they are often misunderstood and can have trouble making and keeping friends. People with ADD need to learn to cope with their disability and to channel their remarkable energy in a positive direction to succeed. Albert Einstein is just one of the famous people said to have had ADD who has made wonderful contributions to the world.

A "multimodal" approach is recommended for treating ADD. This may involve parent participation in behavior modification techniques, an individualized educational program, individual and family counseling, and medication when required.

If you think that you or your child may have an attention deficit, it is important to consult a specialist (a psychologist or psychiatrist who understands ADD and how to treat it) to get a clear diagnosis.

Many other problems may accompany the disorder, so how the ADD is treated often depends on what other conditions are present.

If you need more information about attention deficit disorders, call or write to CH.A.D.D. (Children and Adults with Attention Deficit Disorders). This national, nonprofit organization is dedicated to helping children and adults with ADD succeed. To find a chapter in your area, call the national headquarters at (954) 587-3700 or (800) 233-4050, or write to CH.A.D.D. at 499 Northwest 70th Avenue, Suite 101, Plantation, FL 33317.

Whether you have an attention disorder or not, the following natural methods have been used very successfully in improving concentration levels.

→ ACUPRESSURE ←

Acupressure can be used very effectively to improve your ability to concentrate. It has been found that tension in the shoulders and neck areas can seriously inhibit concentration and cause poor memory, headaches, dizziness, and mental stress, so it is important to keep good blood circulation in these areas.

Using acupressure on the following points for 1 to 2 minutes daily will not only help to improve these symptoms listed, it will also improve mental clarity. The points are easy for children to learn and can be made part of a daily routine. While your children are stimulating these points on themselves, you can do the same.

Be sure to stimulate the points on both sides of your body or directly on the midline of your body. They can be done while sitting or lying down.

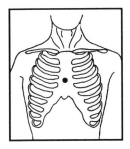

STERNUM POINT
(Conception Vessel 17)

Located one hand's width up from the bottom of the sternum.

Benefits:
Useful for concentration, clear thinking, depression, and anxiety.

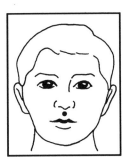

LIP POINT
(Governing Vessel 26)

Just below the nose on the upper lip.

Benefits:
Useful for concentration, dizziness, and memory.

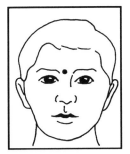

THIRD EYE POINT
(Yin-tang)

Located just between the eyebrows, on the midline of the face.

Benefits:
Useful for concentration, memory, and a positive attitude.

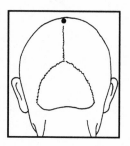

TOP OF HEAD POINT
(Governing Vessel 20)

On midline of top of head, in direct line above ears.

Benefits:
Useful for concentration, headaches, and memory.

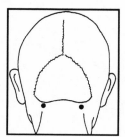

BASE OF SKULL POINT
(Gallbladder 20)

In the hollows of the neck about 2 inches out from the midline of the neck.

Benefits:
Useful for concentration, headaches, and memory.

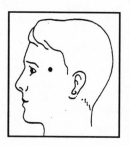

TEMPLE POINT
(Sun Point)

Between outer point of eyebrows and top of ears.

Benefits:
Useful for concentration, headaches, memory, dizziness, and mental stress.

➔ AROMATHERAPY ◄

Since you or your child are often working or out of the house when you need to concentrate, you can place a few drops of the essential oil on a cotton ball and take the aroma with you wherever you go.

Any of these oils can be used to help improve concentration:

➔ **Basil** is useful for headaches and mental fatigue.

➔ **Bay** is good for an overactive mind.

➔ **Cumin** is used for headaches and as a stimulant.

➔ **Dill** helps for headaches and nervousness.

➔ **Rosemary** helps for headaches and fatigue and improves memory.

➔ AYURVEDA ◄

According to the Ayurvedic system of health, good mental function is composed of three attributes: the acquisition, the retention, and the recollection of knowledge.

If you cannot concentrate because you feel tired, this may be a Kapha imbalance, and some Kapha tea may prove stimulating. If you feel you cannot concentrate because you are under stress, some Vata tea may be calming. If you are feeling frustrated with your work, the cooling effects of Pitta tea may help. Both Lisa Marie and her son Freddy take Study Power every day to help with the symptoms of their ADD. College students may want to keep all three teas on hand, particularly during final exams!

→ **Mind Power** is an herbal combination that helps to diminish mental stress. It is recommended for working adults, as it works on improving memory and increasing creativity. It comes in liquid form only.

→ **Study Power** increases general concentration. It is a combination of herbs known for their positive effect on one's ability to concentrate. It strengthens all mental functions, especially comprehension and memory. Study Power comes in tablet form. Adults and children over age 10 should take 1 tablet twice a day; children ages 5 to 10 should take 1 tablet a day.

→ **Youthful Mind,** another herbal combination, is used when you are mentally fatigued. It allows you to focus and relax at the same time. Take these tablets as directed on the bottle.

Ayurveda encourages meditation on a daily basis to help with mental clarity and overall health. Depending on your specific mind/body type, certain kinds of meditation practices may prove more beneficial to you than others.

Vata types derive the most benefit from chanting or from the use of mantras in their meditation.

Pitta types are visually oriented and will enjoy visualization techniques or color meditation.

Kapha types have a strong sense of taste and smell and enjoy using incense or flowers as a part of their meditation.

⤙ **BACH FLOWERS** ⤛

B ach Flowers can be taken on a daily basis, or you may wish to take specific ones as the need arises.

⤙ **Clematis** is for those who are indifferent, inattentive, dreamy, or absentminded. This is the person who withdraws into his or her imagination, whose own creative mind distracts him or her away from reality.

⤙ **Hornbeam** is for those who feel mentally fatigued. These people feel tired even after sleep. They feel that life has become too routine and perk up when something unexpected happens.

⤙ **Impatiens** is for those who feel impatient or irritable. These people feel a mental tension that comes from nervous frustration, a feeling that things are not moving fast enough.

⤙ **Olive** is for those who feel exhausted. Their absence of energy may come from a lack of sleep, a physical illness, a poor diet, or any number of sources. These people are mentally and physically fatigued.

⤙ **Rescue Remedy** is a combination of Bach Flowers that is used for all-purpose emergencies, such as taking a test. Rescue Remedy speeds the healing process when you are recovering from mental turmoil. It can also help to prepare you for upcoming events that may cause you turmoil, such as a job interview or a driving test.

⤙ **White Chestnut** is for those who have persistent unwanted thoughts or who are preoccupied with some worry or episode. These people can't turn off their mind or get an idea out of their heads as much as they would like to.

❧ COLOR THERAPY ❧

Color therapy directly infuses a particular energy vibration into the body to shift its vibratory energy. Specific color energies can significantly improve your ability to concentrate.

Yellow is the color to use to increase concentration. You can use yellow in the following ways:

→ Wear a citrine crystal necklace or citrine earrings. Topaz, amber, and other yellow stones also contain some of the same properties to help concentration. Wear any of these stones every day.

→ Burn a yellow candle for at least 4 hours each day. (Remember: Use caution when burning candles, especially around children and pets.)

→ Sit under a yellow light for 20 minutes each morning.

→ Wear yellow clothing or clothing infused with the vibration of yellow.

→ Take a yellow color bath when you feel scattered or unfocused. Color baths turn your bath water a clear, vivid color. They can be ordered from the Healing Arts Center.

→ Hold something yellow in your left hand while you meditate.

❧ HERBS ❧

To improve concentration, look at the underlying cause that contributes to a lack of concentration. The following herbs are recommended:

→ **Chamomile** is soothing and relaxing. Chamomile comes in capsules or as a tea. Adults may prefer capsules, while children may find the tea, which can be sweetened with honey, preferable.

→ **Valerian root** calms nerves and helps fight stress and anxiety. It comes in capsules or in tea form, although because of the strong taste capsules may be preferred. Valerian is better used for adults and older children.

The following herbs are found only in capsule form. If your child has trouble swallowing them, you can break them open and mix the contents with applesauce or jelly.

→ **Gotu Kola** increases learning ability and memory.

→ **Passionflower** is relaxing.

→ **Skullcap** calms worries.

→ **Thyme** soothes nerves.

→ **Wild Oats** strengthens nerves and is good for mental exhaustion.

→ HOMEOPATHY ←

The following homeopathic remedies are effective in helping to improve concentration:

Baryta carbonica: Used when you feel confused and unable to think clearly.

Iridium: Helps you to concentrate your thinking.

Kali phosphoricum: Used for those times when you feel mentally overworked.

Onosmodium: Used when you feel you lack the power to concentrate and your coordination is poor.

Skatol: Used when you cannot concentrate and you have become depressed by it.

Terebinth: Used when you are unable to concentrate because you are too tired.

→ MEDITATION ←

Meditation is an important part of teaching the mind to concentrate. It also helps people relax so that concentration becomes easier. If you are having trouble meditating, you can use the Bach Flower remedies given in this chapter to help quiet the mind and turn off any inner conflict that may be getting in your way.

Burning a blue or green candle calms the environment and prepares the atmosphere for meditation. White candles provide protection from negative thoughts. Lavender candles foster a spiritual state of mind.

Color meditation involves using the mind to open each chakra, or energy center, in our body and filling it with its natural color for peace and balance. This is done with creative visualization. To think of red, picture a red rose in full bloom or a sparkling red ruby. Using this image, focus on the first chakra, at the base of the spine, and fill it up with the energy of red. Continue this process up through all seven chakras. Here are the chakras and the colors associated with them:

→ **Base of spine:** red (think red rose, ruby, apple)
→ **Top of lumbar:** orange (think marigold, orange, sunset)
→ **Solar plexus:** yellow (think daffodil, topaz, lemon)
→ **Heart:** green (think clover, emerald, pine tree)

→ **Throat:** blue (think sky, lake, sapphire)

→ **Forehead:** indigo (think night sky, iris)

→ **Top of head:** violet (think amethyst, violets)

We have produced a tape called "Color Meditations: For Adults, For Children" that contains two color meditations for adults and three shorter meditations for children. Listening to a guided meditation is an easy way to get started meditating. We've found that this tape helps children to relax and fall asleep at night. "Color Meditations" is available through the Healing Arts Center. (See Appendix 2.)

Some herb tea can help settle the mind and get you ready for meditation. Chamomile is always good, and valerian is relaxing; just make sure that you're not sleepy or it will put you right out! After your meditation, herb tea can help to ground you and bring you back to earth a little bit. Cinnamon-apple or orange spice teas are particularly good for this.

It seems to be more difficult to meditate when you're sick or not feeling well. It is just harder to forget about the aches and pains of the physical body and get into that state of focused concentration. Homeopathic remedies can help in such situations. Look at the homeopathic remedies offered in this chapter to assist you when you meditate.

→ YOGA ←

The following five yogic postures will help in mental concentration and help balance the nervous system.

To improve concentration, we recommend that you and/or your

child do any or all of these postures, three times a week. While they can be done at any time of the day, if you do them in the morning, you will benefit throughout the day.

KING OF DANCER'S POSE
(described on page 69)

PALM TREE POSE

Basic position:

Stand with your feet 4 to 6
inches apart and your arms comfortably
at your sides. Distribute the weight
of your body evenly on both feet.

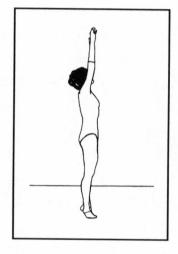

Instructions:

→ Raise your arms over your head with
   your fingers reaching upward.

→ Look at your hands.

→ Slowly rise up onto your toes and completely stretch your whole body.

→ Hold the asana as long as you wish.

→ Slowly return to your original position.

→ Repeat between three and five times.

Breathing:

Inhale as you stretch up.

Hold your breath during your final stretch.

Exhale as you return to your original position.

Benefits:

Strengthens the back, stomach, legs, and feet; helps develop balance, concentration, and correct posture.

ONE-LEG STAND

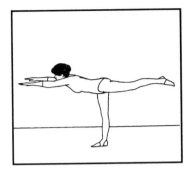

Basic Position:

Stand straight with your feet together.
Raise your arms over your head with
your fingers together.

Instructions:

→ Slowly lean forward, keeping your arms,
  head, and body in a straight line. Simultaneously raise your left leg and
  stretch it backward.
→ Keep your leg in a straight line with the rest of your body. Your body
  should rotate from the right hip joint.
→ The asana is attained when the arms, head, body, and left leg are in one
  straight horizontal line. The right leg should be straight and vertical.
→ Remain in the posture for as long as you comfortably can.
→ Slowly return to the starting position.
→ Repeat the movement using the other leg.
→ Repeat three times on each side.

Breathing:

Inhale while raising the arms.

Exhale while assuming the final posture.

Breathe normally while in the posture.

Inhale while returning to the starting position.

Benefits:

Aids in balance and concentration; strengthens leg muscles.

HALF-MOON POSE

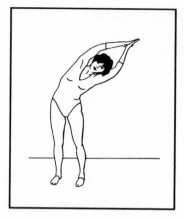

Basic position:

While standing straight with your
arms over your head, interlace your fingers.

Instructions:

→ Slowly bend from your waist as far as
  you can stretch to your left side, then
  slowly return to your original position.
→ Slowly bend to your right side, then slowly return to your original
  position.
→ Try to keep your weight on the balls of your feet as you do this asana.
  This way, you will slowly improve your sense of balance.
→ Bend five times to each side.

Breathing:

Inhale as you stretch your arms over your head.
Exhale as you bend to the side.
Inhale as you straighten up.

Benefits:

Stretches the arms and rib cage; firms the leg muscles.

TREE POSE

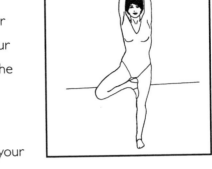

Basic position:

Stand with your feet together and your arms relaxed at your sides. Be sure your weight is distributed evenly between the balls of your feet and your heels.

Instructions:

→ Hold your head straight and focus your eyes on a specific point.

→ Place the sole of your right foot on the inside of your left thigh. You may find it helpful to guide your foot into position with your right hand.

→ When your foot is in place and you feel you have your balance, slowly raise your arms above your head.

→ Place your palms together and straighten your elbows.

→ Continue stretching upward as you hold the position.

→ Hold the posture as long as you comfortably can.

→ Slowly return to the original position.

→ Change legs and repeat.

→ Do the asana three times on each side.

Breathing:

Inhale while establishing the position.

Breathe normally while in the posture.

Exhale while returning to the starting position.

Benefits:

Tones and strengthens the legs; improves balance and concentration; stretches and tones the abdominal organs.

Appendix I

Remedies and Treatments for Various Ailments–Quick Reference

Refer to the List of Illustrations on page vii to locate acupressure point descriptions.

ACNE

Bach Flowers
→ Crab Apple

Color
→ Turquoise

Herbs
→ Aloe vera

Homeopathy
→ Antimonium tartaricum
→ Sulfur

AGITATION

Acupressure
→ 2nd Upper Back Point

ARM PAIN

Acupressure
→ Wrist Point

ASTHMA

Acupressure
→ 2nd Upper Back Point

Bach Flowers
→ Agrimony

BACKACHE

Acupressure
→ Behind the Knee Point

BEDWETTING

Bach Flowers
→ Cherry Plum

Herbs
→ Bearberry

Homeopathy
→ Pulsatilla

BITES

Aromatherapy

+ Lavender
+ Thyme

Bach Flowers

+ Star of Bethlehem

Color

+ Turquoise

Homeopathy

+ Apis mellifica
+ Hepar sulphuris calcareum
+ Ledum palustre

BLISTERS

Aromatherapy

+ Geranium

Color

+ Blue

BODY ACHE

Acupressure

+ Arch Point

BOREDOM

Acupressure

+ 2nd Upper Back Point

BREATHING, DIFFICULTY

Acupressure

+ Wrist Point

BRUISES

Aromatherapy

+ Chamomile
+ Lavender
+ Geranium

Color

+ Blue

Herbs

+ Calendula
+ St. John's Wort

Homeopathy

+ Arnica montana
+ Ledum palustre

BURNS

Aromatherapy
→ Lavender

Ayurveda
→ Pitta Routine
→ Ghee

Color
→ Blue

Herbs
→ St. John's Wort

Homeopathy
→ Cantharis
→ Hypericum

CHICKEN POX

Aromatherapy
→ Chamomile

Homeopathy
→ Antimonium tartaricum
→ Pulsatilla
→ Rhus toxicodendron

CHILLS

Acupressure
→ 1st Upper Back Point
→ 2nd Top of Foot Point

COLD

Acupressure
→ Behind the Knee Point

COLD FEET

Acupressure
→ Arch Point
→ Bottom of Foot Point
→ Ankle Point

COLD SORES

Color
→ Turquoise

Homeopathy
→ Rhus toxicodendron

COLIC

Homeopathy
→ Aconitum napellus
→ Belladonna
→ Chamomilla
→ Magnesium phosphorica

CONGESTION

Acupressure

→ 2nd Upper Back Point
→ Bottom of Foot Point
→ Ankle Point

COUGH

Acupressure

→ 2nd Upper Back Point

CUTS

Aromatherapy

→ Lavender

DIARRHEA

Acupressure

→ Arch Point

DISORIENTATION

Acupressure

→ 2nd Top of Foot Point

EARACHE

Aromatherapy

→ Lavender
→ Tea tree oil

Color

→ Blue

Herbs

→ Mullein Flower

Homeopathy

→ Aconitum napellus
→ Belladonna
→ Chamomilla
→ Ferrum phosphoricum
→ Mercurius vivus
→ Pulsatilla

EAR INFECTION

Aromatherapy

→ Lavender
→ Tea tree oil
→ Thyme

Bach Flowers

→ Crab Apple

Color Therapy

→ Blue

ENERGY, LACK OF

Acupressure

→ Bottom of Foot Point

→ Ankle Point

FATIGUE

Acupressure

→ 1st Top of Foot Point

FEAR

Acupressure

→ Ankle Crease Point

FEVER

Acupressure

→ 1st Upper Back Point

→ Arch Point

Ayurveda

→ Pitta Routine

FLU

Acupressure

→ 1st Upper Back Point

GROWING PAINS

Bach Flowers

→ Walnut

Homeopathy

→ Calcarea phosphorica

HIVES

Homeopathy

→ Rhus toxicodendron

HYPERACTIVITY

Herbs

→ Melissa

→ Passionflower

INFECTION

Aromatherapy

→ Chamomile

Ayurveda

→ Pitta Routine

Bach Flowers

→ Crab Apple

Color Therapy

→ Green

KNEE PAIN

Acupressure

→ Behind the Knee Point

LEG PAIN

Acupressure

→ Behind the Knee Point

MEASLES

Herbs

→ Chamomile

MUMPS

Color

→ Blue

MUSCLES: CRAMPS, SORENESS, WEAKNESS

Acupressure

→ 1st Top of Foot Point

Homeopathy

→ Arnica montana
→ Rhus toxicodendron

PAIN

Herbs

→ Passionflower

RASHES

Ayurveda

→ Ghee

Bach Flowers

→ Crab Apple

RIVALRY, SIBLING

Bach Flowers

→ Holly

SKIN IRRITATION

Ayurveda

→ Refer to Ayurveda section in Chapter 6 for details

Bach Flowers

→ Crab Apple

Color

→ Blue

Herbs

→ Aloe vera

SLEEPLESSNESS

Herbs

→ Chamomile

Homeopathy

→ Calms Forte

SPASMS

Acupressure

→ 1st Top of Foot Point
→ Behind the Knee Point

SPRAIN

Color

→ Blue

Homeopathy

→ Ledum palustre
→ Ruta graveolens

STINGS

Bach Flowers

→ Star of Bethlehem

Color

→ Turquoise

Homeopathy

→ Hypericum
→ Ledum palustre

STOMACH, UPSET

Acupressure

→ Arch Point
→ 2nd Top of Foot Point
→ Ankle Crease Point

Herbs

→ Chamomile

STRESS

Homeopathy

→ Calms Forte

SUNBURN

Color

→ Blue

Homeopathy

→ Cantharis

SWELLING

Homeopathy

→ Apis mellifica

TEETHING

Aromatherapy

→ Chamomile

Bach Flowers

→ Walnut

Homeopathy

→ Calcarea phosphorica

→ Chamomilla

THROAT, SORE

Acupressure

→ Bottom of Foot Point

Aromatherapy

→ Chamomile

TONSILLITIS

Aromatherapy

→ Chamomile

Herbs

→ Chamomile

TOOTHACHE

Homeopathy

→ Chamomilla

WARTS

Color

→ Green

→ Violet

Herbs

→ Thuja leaf oil

WEAK FEET

Acupressure

→ 1st Top of Foot Point

WRIST PAIN

Acupressure

→ Wrist Point

Appendix 2

Resources

All of the products listed in this book are available through

The Healing Arts Center
20315 Ventura Boulevard, Suite C
Woodland Hills, CA 91364
(818) 887-9622

↪ Other sources to contact:

Acupressure Institute
1533 Shattuck Avenue
Berkeley, CA 94709
(415) 845-1058
(800) 442-2232

American Aromatherapy
  Association
PO Box 1222
Fair Oaks, CA 95628

American Association of
  Homeopathic Pharmacies
PO Box 2273
Falls Church, VA 22042
(703) 532-3237

American Association
  of Naturopathic Physicians
2366 Eastlake Avenue East
Seattle, WA 98102
(206) 323-7610

American Chiropractic
  Association
1916 Wilson Boulevard
Suite 300
Arlington, VA 22201
(703) 276-8800

American Osteopathic
  Association
142 East Ontario Street
Chicago, IL 60611
(312) 280-5800

Center for Attention Disorders
2750 Sycamore Drive
Simi Valley, CA 93065
(805) 527-9414

The Chopra Center for Well-Being
7630 Fay Street
La Jolla, CA 92038
(619) 551-7788

CH.A.D.D.
  (Children and Adults with
  Attention Deficit Disorders)
499 Northwest 70th Avenue
Suite 101
Plantation, FL 33317
(954) 587-3700
(800) 233-4050

Maharishi Ayur-Veda
  Medical Center
679 George Hill Road
Lancaster, MA 01523
(508) 365-4549

Maharishi Ayur-Ved Products
  International, Inc.
PO Box 49667
Colorado Springs, CO
80949-9667
(800) 255-8332

Maharishi University of
  Management
Fairfield, IA 52557
(515) 472-5031

National Center For
  Homeopathy
801 North Fairfax Street
Suite 306
Alexandria, VA 22314-1757
(703) 548-7790

Bibliography

Bach, Edward, and F. J. Wheeler. *The Bach Flower Remedy*. New Canaan, Conn.: Keats Publishing, 1977.

Balch, James F., and Phyllis A. Balch. *Prescription for Nutritional Healing*. Garden City, N.Y.: Avery Publications Group, 1990.

Buckland, Raymond. *Practical Color Magick*. St. Paul, Minn.: Llewellyn Publications, 1983.

Castleman, Michael. *Cold Cures*. New York: Fawcett Columbine, 1992.

Chancellor, Philip M. *Bach Flower Remedies*. New Canaan, Conn.: Keats Publishing, 1971.

Chopra, Deepak. *Perfect Health: The Complete Mind/Body Guide*. New York: Harmony Books, 1991.

Dass, Ram. *The Only Dance There Is*. New York: Archer Books, 1974.

Davis, Patricia. *Aroma Therapy: An A-Z*. Woodstock, N.Y.: Beekman Publishers, 1988.

Ferrara, Peter L. *Natural Remedies*. New York: Pinnacle Books, 1984.

Frawley, David. *Ayurvedic Healing*. Salt Lake City, Utah: Passage Press, 1989.

Garion-Hutchings, Nigel and Susan. *The New Concise Guide to Homeopathy*. Rockport, Mass.: Element, Inc., 1995.

Gibbons, De Lamar. *The Self-Help Way to Treat Colitis and Other IBS Conditions*. New Canaan, Conn.: Keats Publishing, 1992.

Gottleib, Bill, ed. *The Doctor's Book of Home Remedies for Children*. Emmaus, Pa.: Rodale Press, 1994.

Hallowell, Edward, and John J. Ratey. *Driven to Distraction*. New York: Pantheon Books, 1994.

Hobbs, Christopher. *Handbook for Herbal Healing: A Concise Guide to Herbal Products*. Capitola, Calif.: Botanica Press, 1990.

Horvilleur, Alain. *The Family Guide to Homeopathy*. Arlington, Va.: Health and Homeopathy Publications, 1989.

Keith, Velma J., and Monteen Gordon. *The How to Herb Book*. Pleasant Grove, Utah: Mayfield Publications, 1982.

Mahesh, Maharishi, trans. *Bhagavad-Gita*. New York: Penguin Books, 1990.

Muramoto, Naboru. *Healing Ourselves*. New York: Avon Books, 1973.

Panos, Maesimund B., and Jane Heimlich. *Homeopathic Medicine at Home*. New York: Putnam Books, 1980.

Rose, Barry. *The Family Health Guide to Homeopathy*. Berkeley, Calif.: Celestial Arts, 1993.

Scheffer, Mechthild. *Bach Flower Therapy: Theory and Practice*. Rochester, Vt.: Healing Arts Press, 1988.

Stewart, Mary, and Kathy Phillips. *Yoga for Children*. New York: Simon & Schuster, 1992.

Strohecker, James. *Alternative Medicine: The Definitive Guide*. Puyallup, Wash.: Future Medicine Publishing, 1994.

Taylor, Louise. *Acupressure, Yoga and You*. New York: Japan Publications, 1984.

———*Ki: Energy for Everybody*. New York: Japan Publications, 1990.

———*Simple Ways to Wellness*. Boston: Charles E. Tuttle Co., Inc., 1995.

———*A Woman's Book of Yoga*. Boston: Charles E. Tuttle Co., Inc., 1993.

Tenny, Louise. *Health Handbook*. Pleasant Grove, Utah: Woodland Books, 1994.

Ullman, Dana. *Homeopathic Medicine for Children and Infants*. Los Angeles: Jeremy P. Tarcher Inc., 1992.

Valent, Jean. *The Practice of Aroma Therapy*. Rochester, Vt.: Healing Arts Press, 1980.

Vickery, Donald M., and James F. Fries. *Take Care of Yourself*. Reading, Mass.: Addison-Wesley, 1990.

Wallace, Amy, and Bill Henkin. *The Psychic Healing Book*. Berkeley Calif.: Wingbow Press, 1985.

Weber, Marcea. *Encyclopedia of Natural Health and Healing for Children*. Rocklin, Calif.: Prima Publishing, 1992.

Weil, Andrew. *Health and Healing*. Boston: Houghton Mifflin, 1985.

Weiner, Michael A., and Kathleen Goss. *Healing Children Naturally*. San Rafael, Calif.: Quantum Books, 1982.

Worwood, Valerie Ann. *The Complete Book of Essential Oils and Aroma Therapy*. San Rafael, Calif.: New World Library, 1991.

Zand, Janet, Rachel Walton, and Bob Roundtree. *Smart Medicine for a Healthier Child*. Garden City, N.Y.: Avery Publications Group, 1994.

About the Authors

Louise Taylor received her master of science degree from California State University, Northridge. She has a doctor of divinity degree from the Universal Life Church. Her studies of Hatha Yoga took her to India, where she gained firsthand impressions of the yogic system. She is a student of Siddha Yoga, and as a devotee of Guru Swami Chidvilasananda, she has practiced yogic disciplines for the past ten years. Ms. Taylor has taught health-oriented courses at Mount Saint Mary's College in Los Angeles; Los Angeles Mission College; California State University, Northridge; and Santa Monica College. In 1984 she founded the Healing Arts Center in Woodland Hills, California, and currently directs this center, where a variety of alternative health practices are taught.

Ms. Taylor is the author of *Acupressure, Yoga and You,* which integrates the benefits of Hatha Yoga and acupressure; *Ki: Energy for Everybody,* a look at ways to improve the body and increase your energy from both the Eastern and Western perspectives; *A Woman's Book of Yoga,* which is a workbook for Yoga practice; and *Simple Ways to Wellness,* a guide to using acupressure, affirmations, imagery, and color therapy for self-healing. Ms. Taylor has developed a cassette tape, "Color Meditations: for Adults, for Children," which guides its listeners into peaceful, stress-free meditations as well as balancing the powerful chakra energy centers.

Lisa Marie Nelson is an award-winning producer and songwriter in the children's entertainment industry. She has created products in nearly every medium, including the Positive Music for Today's Kids series of audiotapes and CDs and the Karate for Kids series of home videos. Her music videos for children have aired on Nickelodeon and The Learning Channel. She is the author of *Freddy Bear's Wakeful Winter,* a children's story of an active little bear who refuses to hibernate. Ms. Nelson has appeared on national television many times to discuss her Positive Parenting philosophy.

After studying alternative healing treatments and techniques for many years at the Healing Arts Center in Woodland Hills, California, Ms. Nelson now teaches classes there. She works with many nonprofit groups to help children, including ChildHelp USA and the Starlight Foundation. She serves on the board of directors for CH.A.D.D. of the Conejo Valley. Ms. Nelson holds a degree in sociology from the University of California, Los Angeles, and a doctorate of philosophy in religion from the Universal Life Church.